Solutions from My Ancestors for Everyday Health Problems

JUANITA HOLADAY

DEDICATION

My intention is to share the information that was passed down to me from my family generation by generation. My hope is that you, the reader, will be able to find this information as valuable as I have, as well as those who have benefited greatly from these sacred secrets.

I have tried to bring them up to speed so that they have meaningful application in a world that has progressed in a manner that could have been better, if we embraced these primitive technologies, rather than pharmaceutical treatments.

CONTENTS

INTRODUCTION

As a child, I watched in awe as the elders in my family prepared remedies for all kinds of ailments—using plants, oils, and even simple prayers. They didn't just treat symptoms; they understood the body as an interconnected system and believed that healing required balance—of the body, the mind, and the spirit. Little did I know, these moments of observation would plant the seeds for a lifelong journey into the world of natural healing.

The knowledge shared by my family wasn't written in textbooks or taught in classrooms. It was passed down through stories, traditions, and rituals—a living connection to the wisdom of our ancestors. My grandmother would pick herbs from her garden, my uncle would mix teas, and my mother would soothe our ailments with her hands and an unshakable faith in the healing power of nature. This legacy became the foundation of my work as a holistic healer and, ultimately, this book.

Solutions from My Ancestors for Everyday Health Problems is a labor of love, born from the understanding that the wisdom of the past is still profoundly relevant today. At a time when our fast-paced, modern lives often leave us disconnected from nature and ourselves, this book invites you to slow down, listen, and rediscover the healing tools that have always been available to us.

The goal of this book is not to reject modern medicine but to provide an empowering complement to it. There are moments when pharmaceuticals and medical interventions are essential, even life-saving. Yet, there is also a space for natural remedies—practices that address the root causes of our discomfort rather than simply masking the symptoms. Herbs, botanicals, mindfulness practices, and energy healing have been used for centuries to bring the body back into balance, and they remain as effective as ever.

This book is a bridge between ancient wisdom and contemporary challenges. Each chapter explores different facets of natural healing, from understanding the messages your body is sending you, to exploring herbs and botanicals, to learning how your thoughts and emotions influence your physical health. It also addresses the ways our modern lifestyles, diets, and habits can disconnect us from our natural state of well-being—and how we can find our way back.

I've woven my personal experiences into these pages, sharing both the triumphs and the lessons learned along the way. My intention is to honor the sacred knowledge of my ancestors while making it accessible and practical for you in today's world.

Whether you're seeking alternatives to medications, looking to deepen your connection with your body, or simply curious about how natural remedies can enrich your life, this book is for you. It's my hope that it will serve as a guide, a companion, and an inspiration as you embark on your own journey toward natural wellness.

May these pages remind you of the powerful connection we all share with the earth, with our ancestors, and with each other. And may you find healing, balance, and strength in the timeless solutions offered by the wisdom of the past.

Contact me at juanitaholaday.com for more information.

1 WHAT IS GOING ON WITH YOUR BODY?

Have you ever wondered why your body reacts the way it does, or why certain things, like fatigue, aches, or even sudden health changes, seem to appear out of nowhere? Our bodies are always sending us signals—sometimes loud and clear, and other times subtle, like a whisper. I've learned that paying attention to these signals is one of the most important things we can do for our health.

In this chapter, we'll explore the fascinating ways our bodies work and why they sometimes struggle. From understanding how blood clots form and what they mean, to learning about the foods that strengthen or weaken our bones, this chapter dives into how small choices can make a big difference. This isn't about feeling overwhelmed or confused—it's about becoming curious and empowered to listen to your body and care for it with love and intention.

Just like our ancestors, who relied on the wisdom of nature and their keen understanding of the body, we can embrace that same approach today. By blending ancient knowledge with modern insights, we can learn to nurture our health in ways that align with how our bodies are designed to thrive. Let's take this journey together and uncover the answers to what's really going on inside us—and how we can work with our bodies to live our best lives.

What Causes Blood Clots?

What is a Blood Clot?

A blood clot forms when blood thickens into a clump, like a gel. Clots can happen due to an injury or sometimes without any clear reason. Good blood clots help you stop bleeding when you get a cut. But some clots can be dangerous, especially if they move to other parts of your body.

What Can Cause a Dangerous Blood Clot?

Some common causes include:
- Medications
- Heart issues
- Family history of clots
- Sitting or lying down for long times
- Smoking

How to Tell if You Have a Blood Clot

If you get a clot in your leg, it may be swollen, red, and hurt. If you notice this, call your doctor or go to the hospital.

Tips to Prevent Blood Clots

- Move Often: Don't sit too long. Get up, walk around, and keep your blood moving.
- Drink Water: Stay hydrated to help your blood flow.
- Lose Weight: If you're overweight, losing some weight can help.
- Avoid Alcohol: Alcohol can dehydrate you.
- Reduce Stress: High stress can increase your risk of clots.

Blood clots can go away on their own naturally but it takes time, time for the body to break it down and absorb it, but you still need to be careful until you get checked by the doctor to make sure it is gone.

It may take weeks or months, it all depends on your body's healing power.

Take Herbs

If you want to heal with herbs then you need to take the following herbs to help your body to heal.

- Turmeric
- Ginkgo biloba
- Ginger
- Cassia cinnamon
- Cayenne peppers
- Garlic

these are just a few that can help keep in dissolving blood clots and keeping them from forming.

And there are many more herbs that can help.

It takes time for the body to heal itself and with natural herbs the body responds better to the natural herb then the synthetic drugs.

Osteoporosis Stop Eating Foods that Dissolve Bones

Many of us enjoy foods that add flavor and variety to our meals, but some of these can be harmful to our bones over time. Certain foods actually cause our bones to lose calcium, which can lead to weaker bones and worsen osteoporosis. Here are seven foods to limit or avoid if you want to protect your bone health.

1. Soda

Soda contains phosphorus, an element that can cause your body to lose calcium, which is crucial for strong bones. Regularly drinking soda can increase bone loss over time, making bones more fragile. If you enjoy soda, try to drink it less often, and consider adding more calcium-rich foods like milk or yogurt to your diet to support your bones.

2. Salt

Many processed foods are high in salt, which makes them tasty but can cause your body to lose calcium. When you eat too much salt, your kidneys excrete more calcium, meaning less is available to keep your bones strong. Look at food labels for sodium content, especially in packaged foods, and aim to reduce salt intake by preparing more home-cooked meals.

3. Beans

Beans are a healthy source of fiber and protein but contain a compound called phytates that can interfere with calcium absorption. Phytates bind to calcium and prevent it from being fully absorbed in the body. Soaking beans before cooking can help reduce phytate levels, allowing you to enjoy the benefits of beans without losing bone-strengthening calcium.

4. Alcohol

While moderate alcohol intake may not have a major impact, excessive drinking can reduce bone density. Alcohol interferes with the body's ability to absorb calcium and other nutrients that support bone health. Aim to limit alcohol intake to one or two drinks per day to protect your bones.

5. Caffeine

Caffeine, found in coffee, tea, and some sodas, can also reduce calcium absorption. Although caffeine has some health benefits, it's best to enjoy it in moderation. If you're a coffee drinker, consider keeping it to one or two cups a day, and be sure to include calcium-rich foods in your diet to offset any effects on your bones.

6. Processed Meats

Processed meats like deli cuts, hot dogs, and jerky are often high in sodium and preservatives. The salt content in these meats can interfere with calcium absorption, which is critical for maintaining strong bones. Try to choose fresh meats or reduce your intake of processed meats to limit this effect.

7. Certain Vegetables

Some vegetables, such as tomatoes, potatoes, and peppers, may promote inflammation, which can indirectly affect bones over time. Additionally, leafy greens like spinach and Swiss chard, while rich in calcium, contain oxalates that bind to calcium and make it harder for your body to absorb. Eating these vegetables is still beneficial but enjoy them in balance with other calcium-rich foods.

To support strong bones, eat a variety of nutrient-dense foods, especially those high in calcium and vitamin D, and limit the foods that interfere with bone health. Encouraging a balanced diet for your family and modeling these habits can help everyone build and maintain strong bones.

Why is My Hair Falling Out?

Many people, both men and women, start to lose hair as they get older and wonder, "Why is my hair falling out?" Some people even begin to lose hair at a young age. I once knew a woman who lost all her hair, and the doctor thought it might be because of stress. Stress can cause hair loss, and it's a common reason for hair to fall out.

When hair falls out in small, round patches, this condition is called Alopecia Areata. It can be scary to see patches of hair missing without knowing why. This hair loss can happen on the scalp, eyebrows, eyelashes, or other areas with hair. Sometimes, hair breaks off and grows back but might come in a different color or texture, like thinner or even white.

Common Causes of Hair Loss

There are many reasons why hair falls out, including:

- Genetics (inherited from family)
- Stress
- Smoking
- Pregnancy
- Medications
- Hair coloring or styling
- Diet

If you're losing hair, a doctor can help by checking your hair and doing a blood test to find the cause.

Natural Ways to Help Your Hair Grow

Here are some natural methods that may help:

- Scalp Massage
  - Massaging your scalp each day with your fingers or hair oils can improve blood flow, which may help hair grow. Plus, it's relaxing and can reduce stress!
- Aloe Vera
  - Aloe vera helps with dandruff and clears blocked hair follicles. Using aloe vera shampoo a few times a week can keep your scalp and hair healthy.

- Coconut Oil
  - o Coconut oil is great for hair. Massage it into your scalp and hair. If your hair is dry, leave it in overnight, or leave it in for one to two hours before washing it out.
- Onion Juice
  - o Onion juice can improve blood flow to the scalp and help hair growth for people with Alopecia Areata. Blend an onion, squeeze the juice through a cheesecloth, and apply it to your scalp for 15 minutes before washing it out.
- Rosemary and Cinnamon Water
  - o Boil four sticks of cinnamon in a pot of water for 15 minutes. Add four sprigs of rosemary, simmer for another 20 minutes, and let it cool. Spray it on your scalp, massage, and let it dry.

These natural treatments can be helpful for hair health, but remember, it's also important to keep stress low and have a balanced diet.

What Are Fibroids and What Causes Them?

Have you ever heard of fibroids? I had fibroids years ago and eventually needed surgery to remove them because they were so painful. The pain was so strong that it would wake me up at night. While fibroids sometimes shrink on their own, waiting can be too painful.

What Causes Fibroids?

Fibroids are non-cancerous growths that form in the uterus. They often grow due to hormones, especially estrogen and progesterone. These hormones cause the lining of the uterus to grow each month in preparation for pregnancy. With extra hormones, fibroids can grow bigger, which may lead to problems.

How Fibroids Affect the Body

Fibroids can cause heavy menstrual bleeding, severe cramps, back pain, and even blood clots during your period. The clots form because the fibroids block the blood flow, making it harder for the blood to pass through. If a blood clot is the size of a quarter or larger, it may be a sign that you have many fibroids.

Fibroids can also affect other organs. My fibroids grew so large that I had to have a hysterectomy (removal of the uterus), and they even affected my ovaries and intestines. Every woman is different, and fibroids usually affect women over 40, but younger women can get them too.

Symptoms of Fibroids

Fibroids can make your stomach feel hard or swollen. In some cases, they can press on nearby organs, causing discomfort.

Natural Treatments for Fibroids

There are new medical treatments today, but some people also try natural remedies. Traditional Chinese medicine, for example, uses a mix of herbs called Gui Zhi Fu Ling Tang to balance hormone levels and keep the uterus healthy.

Other natural remedies include:

- Green tea: Helps reduce inflammation.
- Chasteberry: Balances hormones and may help with heavy bleeding and painful periods.

If fibroids are causing you pain, it's a good idea to see your doctor. However, if you want to explore natural options, you might find herbs that can ease the pain and help shrink fibroids over time.

When I was young my mom passed away, I didn't have anyone to talk to about my painful periods, and I wish I had known this information then—it would have been helpful!

Constipation: Not Going When You Need to Go

Have you ever felt sluggish and didn't know why? It may sound simple, but if you aren't having regular bowel movements, that might be the problem.

When we don't go to the bathroom regularly, the food we eat gets stuck in our system and becomes compacted, kind of like when a machine squashes cardboard into small bundles. If we ignore our body's signals to go, it can lead to that uncomfortable feeling of needing to go but not being able to.

Some people can solve constipation by drinking more water and eating foods with fiber. But for others, constipation can become a serious problem, with some people going days or even weeks without a bowel movement.

What Causes Constipation?

Constipation can be caused by many things, such as:

- Medications
- Not drinking enough water
- Ignoring the urge to go
- Lack of exercise
- Not eating enough fiber
- Pregnancy

Our bodies absorb water from the food we eat, but if too much water is absorbed, the stool becomes hard and dry, which makes it difficult to pass.

How to Prevent Constipation

Fiber helps keep your bowel movements regular. All plants and fruits contain fiber, which is important for our digestive system.

Here's how much fiber you need each day:

- Men: 38 grams
- Women: 25 grams
- As we age, the amount decreases to 30 grams for men and 21 grams for women.

Most people don't eat enough fiber, but you can make simple changes to improve this.

Tips to Relieve and Prevent Constipation:

- Eat More Fruits and Vegetables
  - Instead of chips or cookies, choose healthy snacks like apples, carrots, or celery.
- Add Vegetables to Meals
  - Use more vegetables and less meat in meals like stews or stir-fried dishes.
- Stay Hydrated
  - Drink plenty of water. Avoid sugary drinks like soda; try fruit smoothies or natural juices instead.
- Exercise Daily
  - Aim for at least 30 minutes a day of activity to help keep your digestion on track.

By making these small changes, you can help your body stay regular and avoid constipation. Stay active, eat healthy, and drink lots of water to keep everything running smoothly.

Do You Have Problems with Your Prostate?

Many men don't know much about their prostate or what it does. The prostate is a small gland, about the size of a walnut, that's part of the reproductive system. It sits between your bladder and rectum and surrounds the urethra, a tube that carries urine out of your body.

The prostate's main job is to add fluid to semen, which helps sperm travel from the testicles. As men get older, the prostate naturally gets bigger. By age 40, it may be the size of an apricot, and by age 60, it can grow to the size of a lemon.

As the prostate grows, it can press on the urethra, making it harder to urinate or ejaculate. This condition is known as benign prostatic hyperplasia or BPH. Age and family history can increase the chances of developing BPH.

Signs of an Enlarged Prostate

- If your prostate is enlarged, you might notice these signs:

- Your bladder doesn't empty completely when you pee.
- You feel the need to go to the bathroom often.
- You start and stop multiple times while peeing.
- You have to strain to get a steady stream going.

If you notice any of these symptoms, it's important to talk to your doctor. Waiting too long can lead to serious problems with your kidneys or bladder.

Everyone is different; some men don't have many symptoms, but it's still good to let your doctor know. They can keep an eye on it and recommend treatments if needed.

Treatment Options

Your doctor will suggest treatments based on your symptoms and age. If your symptoms are mild, your doctor may just want to monitor you with yearly check-ups. They may also suggest reducing fluids before bedtime and cutting back on caffeine and alcohol.

There are also medications for BPH (Benign Prostatic Hyperplasia), but some may have risks like cancer. If you prefer natural remedies, some herbs might help with symptoms:

- Saw Palmetto
  - This is a popular herb for BPH. It reduces the size of the prostate by blocking a hormone called dihydrotestosterone.
- Stinging Nettle
  - Often combined with Saw Palmetto, it helps reduce inflammation.
- Pumpkin Seeds
  - These contain beta-sitosterol, which can improve urine flow and help empty the bladder.

Helpful Tips for Prostate Health

- Try to use the bathroom before leaving the house.
- Drink two liters of water a day.
- Don't drink water two hours before bedtime.
- Get regular exercise.
- Reduce stress.

Doctors are still researching the exact causes of BPH, but many believe it's due to natural hormonal changes with age. I hope this helps you better understand your prostate health.

The wisdom of traditional teachings often reminds us of the interconnected nature of health and balance. Just as the rivers flow freely when unobstructed, so too should the systems within our bodies. Challenges such as blockages, discomfort, or imbalance serve as signals that our inner harmony requires attention.

Listening to the Body's Signals

Ancient guidance emphasizes observing and understanding the body's subtle messages. Whether it's a sign of discomfort, a shift in function, or a persistent challenge, these are reminders to pause and realign with practices that nurture vitality.

Natural Allies for Healing

Nature offers a treasure trove of remedies to support the body's ability to heal and restore itself. Herbs, natural foods, and mindful practices work gently, addressing root causes rather than masking symptoms. From promoting circulation to soothing inflammation, these natural methods align with the rhythms of the body and the earth.

Balancing Action and Rest

Staying active and maintaining movement reflects the energy of life, but so does the need for rest and regeneration. Movement prevents stagnation, while rest allows the body to heal and strengthen. By weaving these principles together, we can support both prevention and recovery.

Holistic Care for Every Stage

As life progresses, the needs of the body evolve. Adapting to these changes with nurturing habits, mindful nutrition, and an open heart ensures longevity and quality of life. Preventive care, regular attention to well-being, and embracing natural cycles lead to resilience and harmony.

Through intentional living and embracing the gifts of the natural world, we honor the wisdom that our ancestors have passed down. This wisdom reminds us that the path to health lies in balance, awareness, and a deep connection to the earth and its rhythms.

Scabies: What Are They and Where Do They Come From?

Have you ever heard of scabies or known someone who had them? Scabies are caused by tiny mites called *Sarcoptes scabiei*. These mites are so small you can't see them with the naked eye. They burrow under the top layer of skin, lay eggs, and live there.

The most common symptom of scabies is intense itching, often with small, pimple-like sores. Scabies can affect anyone, anywhere in the world, and can spread very quickly.

How Does Scabies Spread?

Scabies spreads through close, skin-to-skin contact, such as sharing bedding, towels, or spending time touching someone's skin. Quick contact, like a handshake or a hug, usually isn't enough to spread scabies. Scabies mites can't jump or fly, and they move very slowly. However, because we enjoy things like cuddling, hugging, and other close contact, the mites can have enough time to spread.

Can You Get Scabies from Pets?

No, humans can't catch scabies from pets, and pets can't get human scabies. Animals can get a similar condition called mange, but it's caused by a different type of mite.

Who is Most at Risk?

People who live or work in close quarters, like:

- Prison inmates
- People in childcare centers
- People in nursing homes or institutional care

If you see someone with crusted, itchy hands, especially between the fingers, it might be a severe case of scabies. This form is very contagious and should be reported right away.

Natural Treatments for Scabies

Some natural treatments may help with scabies:

- Tea Tree Oil
    o This can help kill mites but might not work on eggs. It also reduces itching and helps the skin heal.
- Neem Oil
    o Neem comes from a tree and is available in oils, creams, and soaps. It can help kill both mites and their eggs.
- Aloe Vera
    o Aloe vera gel can ease itching and may help get rid of the mites.

If these treatments don't work, see your doctor. They may prescribe a special cream that you apply all over your body for 24 hours. Sometimes, you may need to reapply it if itching continues.

Even though these mites are tiny, they can cause a lot of trouble. Remember, sometimes the smallest things in life can be the hardest to deal with!

Eyebrow and Eyelash Lice

Have you ever heard of eye lice or eyebrow lice? The medical name for these tiny bugs is Phthiriasis Palpebrarum, and while they are rare, they do happen, especially with the rise in eyelash extensions.

Eye lice are actually a type of pubic lice that can spread to the eyes. They can get there when lice from other parts of the body (like the pubic area) transfer through contact with your hands. If you touch those areas and then touch your eyes, lice can latch onto your lashes. This is a great reminder to always wash your hands!

The Life Cycle of Eye Lice

Here's what happens after lice attach to your lashes:

- Eggs (nits) hatch in about 6-10 days.
- The lice grow into adults within 2-3 weeks.
- Adult lice live for another 3-4 weeks, and each one lays about 30 eggs.

If you find eye lice, check other areas with coarse hair, like your eyebrows, armpits, and pubic hair, to see if they've spread.

Symptoms of Eye Lice

Here are some signs that you may have eye lice:

- Intense itching at the base of your eyelashes, often worse at night.
- Sticky eyelashes.
- Redness or tearing in the eyes.
- A tickling feeling.
- Small brown or black spots at the base of the lashes.

Sometimes itching around the eyes could be caused by dry skin or an allergy to eyebrow wax or other skin products. But if itching continues, it could be lice.

How to Avoid Eye Lice

To help prevent eye lice:

- Don't share personal items like brushes, bedding, scarves, or hats.

- If you think you have eye lice, you can try applying a little petroleum jelly on your eyelashes for 30 minutes, twice a day, for three days. This may help kill the lice.

- Aloe vera may also be soothing.

If you're not sure, it's best to see your doctor to check for lice or possible allergies.

Prevention is the best way to protect yourself. Washing your hands regularly and avoiding shared items can make a big difference. Reading about lice may make you feel itchy, but don't worry—just stay cautious and clean.

Healing Through Natural Wisdom

For generations, natural remedies have been trusted to restore balance and alleviate discomfort. The properties of plants and oils, carefully harvested and applied, serve as gentle but effective solutions. They not only address immediate concerns but also support the body's ability to heal and protect itself.

Practices of Prevention and Care

Mindful practices, like regular cleansing and avoiding shared personal items, align with age-old teachings that emphasize purity and self-awareness. By respecting our surroundings and nurturing cleanliness, we honor our bodies and create a protective barrier against unwanted disruptions.

Lessons from the Small and Unseen

These experiences teach resilience and the importance of staying attuned to subtle changes in our environment. Even the smallest discomfort can lead to greater wisdom when approached with patience and care.

Through awareness, natural remedies, and preventive habits, we can maintain harmony and well-being, drawing upon the enduring lessons of interconnectedness and self-care that ancient cultures have long cherished.

Difference Between Nearsighted and Farsighted

People often mix up nearsightedness and farsightedness. Here's how to tell the difference:

Farsightedness (Hyperopia)

If you're farsighted, you can see objects clearly when they're far away, but things up close look blurry. This happens because light entering the eye focuses behind the retina instead of directly on it.

Causes of farsightedness include:

- A shorter-than-normal eyeball
- A flatter or less round lens

Farsightedness can make it hard to read or see things clearly up close, like books, smartphones, or even your dinner plate. It is often genetic, meaning it runs in families.

Nearsightedness (Myopia)

If you're nearsighted, you can see nearby objects clearly, but things far away look blurry. This happens when light entering the eye focuses in front of the retina instead of directly on it.

Causes of nearsightedness include:

- An eyeball that is longer than normal
- A lens that is more curved than usual

This makes it difficult to see faraway objects, like a whiteboard at school, road signs, or anything else at a distance. Like farsightedness, nearsightedness is often genetic.

How Glasses and Contact Lenses Help

Corrective lenses (glasses or contacts) help fix both nearsightedness and farsightedness by bending the light to focus directly on the retina. However, glasses and contacts are temporary fixes—when you take them off, your vision goes back to its original state.

Eye Care Tips for Everyone

Our eyes do a lot of work every day, especially if we spend a lot of time looking at screens. Here are some ways to care for them:

- Take Short Breaks

- o If you're using a computer or looking at a screen, take a break every 20 minutes. Look at something far away, blink a few times to moisten your eyes, and give your eyes a chance to relax. This can help prevent eye strain and dryness.

- Limit Screen Time
  - o Try to limit how much time you spend staring at screens. Looking at screens can tire your eyes and sometimes make them red, dry, or irritated.

- Blink Often
  - o Blinking keeps your eyes moist and can help prevent dryness, especially when you're using a screen for a long time.

Natural Remedies to Support Eye Health

There are some natural herbs that may support eye health. These herbs have been used for many years as traditional remedies:

- Fennel
  - o Fennel is rich in vitamins A and C, which are good for eye health. You can make a tea with fennel seeds or use a fennel eye wash. These nutrients can help keep your eyes healthy over time.

- Passionflower
  - o Passionflower is known to relax the blood vessels around the eyes, improving blood flow and reducing eye strain. Drinking passionflower tea or using it in supplement form may be soothing for tired eyes.

- Ginkgo Biloba
  - o This ancient herb is believed to improve circulation around the eyes, ensuring that blood flows well in the area. Good circulation helps keep eyes healthy and prevents eye strain. Ginkgo Biloba is usually taken as a supplement.

Giving Your Eyes a Rest

Unlike other body parts, our eyes are constantly working, even when the rest of us is resting. We use our eyes to look at phones, computers, TVs, and more, giving them very little downtime.

Try these simple exercises to give your eyes a break:

- Palming
    - Rub your hands together to warm them up, then gently place your palms over your closed eyes. Relax and breathe deeply for a minute. This warmth can feel soothing for tired eyes.

- 20-20-20 Rule
    - Every 20 minutes, look at something 20 feet away for 20 seconds. This can help prevent eye strain from close-up work.

Remember, healthy habits and natural remedies can support good eye health, but it's also important to see an eye doctor if you have any vision concerns.

Color Blindness: Are We Born With It?

Did you know that some people are color blind and may not even know it? For them, the way they see colors feels completely normal.

Our eyes have three types of color-detecting cells called cones, which send color signals to our brain. However, some people are missing one type of cone or have a faulty cone, which leads to color blindness. This condition affects about 8% of men worldwide but only about 0.5% of women.

Types of Color Blindness

Red-Green Color Blindness

People with normal color vision, called trichromats, see all colors because they have all three types of cones. However, if one type of cone doesn't work correctly, they become dichromats, meaning they see fewer color combinations—around 10,000 instead of the millions that trichromats see.

The most common form is red-green color blindness, which mostly affects men because it's linked to the X chromosome. Men have only one X chromosome, so if the color vision gene on it is faulty, they are more likely to be color blind.

- Protanomaly
    - People have a weaker sensitivity to red light.
- Deuteranomaly

o   People have a weaker sensitivity to green light.

Both make it difficult to see reds, greens, and oranges clearly but make blues and yellows easier to see.

Blue-Yellow Color Blindness

Tritanomaly affects the blue cone, making it hard to tell blue from green and yellow from violet. This type is rare, affecting about 1 in 30,000 to 50,000 people.

Total Color Blindness

Achromatopsia is a rare form of color blindness where people see only black, white, and shades of gray because they don't have any functioning cones. This condition affects about 1 in 33,000 people.

What Causes Color Blindness?

Color blindness can be caused by:

- Genetics (inherited from parents)
- Illness
- Medications
- Chemical exposure
- Accidents

At this time, there is no cure for color blindness, but it's a good idea to check young children, around ages 3 to 5, for color vision issues before they start school. Just because it's called color blindness doesn't mean they can't see; they just see colors differently.

Challenges with Color Blindness

People who are color blind might find it hard to choose clothes or pick ripe fruit, as they may see colors in shades of gray, similar to old black-and-white movies. Teaching kids with color blindness simple tricks to recognize colors, like looking for specific marks on fruit, can help them manage.

If you became color blind as an adult, do you think it would be hard to adjust?

The wonders of human perception remind us how each individual experiences the world uniquely. From the clarity of vision to the way we interpret colors, these experiences shape how we engage with and navigate our surroundings. Just as nature's wisdom has taught us to value balance and adaptability, so too can these principles guide us in nurturing and protecting our sight.

Understanding and Supporting Vision

When challenges arise, such as blurred vision or difficulty distinguishing colors, they are opportunities to deepen our awareness and care for our eyes. With tools ranging from ancient herbal remedies to mindful practices, we can embrace a holistic approach to maintaining and enhancing our vision.

Listening to Our Eyes

The eyes, like the rest of our body, communicate their needs. Whether it's the strain from modern technology or the subtle shifts in perception over time, these signals are reminders to rest, nourish, and tend to this vital sense. Simple practices like taking breaks, focusing on distant objects, or enjoying natural remedies can make a meaningful difference.

Seeing Beyond the Physical

Even in the face of unique challenges like color perception differences, individuals find ways to adapt and thrive. These experiences teach resilience and innovation, offering lessons that echo the adaptability found in nature.

By honoring the health of our eyes and celebrating the diverse ways people perceive the world, we connect more deeply with the wisdom of nature and the gifts of sight. Through care and mindfulness, we can ensure that this precious sense continues to guide us through life's vibrant landscapes.

2 MODERN ISSUES

Have you ever stopped to think about what's really in the products we use every day or the food we eat? Modern life has made many things easier, but it's also filled our world with chemicals and hidden ingredients that we rarely question. I know I didn't always look closely at labels or wonder how certain products might affect my health over time. But the more I learned, the more I realized how important it is to understand what we're putting into our bodies and onto our skin.

Every day, we make choices without realizing their long-term effects. From the lotions we apply to the food we trust to be safe, we often assume these things are harmless. But as I dug deeper into the science and history behind modern products, I discovered that many contain ingredients that may do more harm than good. How did we stray so far from the natural ways that kept our ancestors healthy?

This chapter is about shining a light on those hidden ingredients and learning to make more informed choices. Modern living comes with challenges, but it also offers opportunities to learn from the wisdom of the past. Whether it's exploring natural alternatives or taking small steps to avoid harmful products, we have the power to support our bodies in better ways. Together, let's explore how to navigate these modern issues with a mix of awareness, ancient wisdom, and practical solutions. When we know better, we can live healthier, more natural lives.

FDA Approved? Look Inside

Do herbs still work well in our bodies after years of using products filled with chemicals? Over time, we've come to rely on many items that may contain hidden, potentially harmful ingredients. Think about the products you use every day:

- Lotions
- Hair colors
- Nail polish
- Processed foods

Our food is often treated with pesticides and chemicals to keep bugs away, and sometimes these chemicals are listed under different names that make them hard to recognize. Unless you know what these names mean, it's easy to miss them.

Here's an example: A man who worked with turpentine—a chemical used to thin paint—was surprised to find it listed as an ingredient in his kids' breakfast cereal, but under a different name. He realized his children were unknowingly eating something he used for industrial work.

FDA Approved? "WOW!"

We trust the FDA to check our food and products for safety, but harmful ingredients sometimes slip through. If a parent was caught poisoning a child, they would likely go to jail. But companies are often able to continue using questionable ingredients with only minor consequences. This is why it's important for us to pay attention to what we eat, drink, and put on our skin.

Our skin is like a sponge that absorbs everything we put on it. Here's a look at some common products and their ingredients:

- Lotions
  - Many lotions contain formaldehyde, a preservative also used to keep dead bodies from decaying.
- Hair Color
  - Hair dyes often contain ammonia, which opens the hair cuticle so it can take in color. They also use peroxide, which changes the pH of hair, allowing it to lighten.
- Nail Polish
  - Nail polish is made with nitrocellulose, a flammable and sometimes explosive ingredient. Breathing in nail polish

fumes over time can have health effects, especially with regular, long-term exposure.

These products may make us look nice, but they also come with risks. Your body may eventually show signs that it's had enough, like persistent itching, rashes, or other reactions. These are signals that something might be wrong. Ignoring these warnings could lead to lasting health issues.

Can Herbs Help Undo the Damage?

If you've used these chemical-laden products for years, you may wonder if natural remedies can reverse the damage. I believe they can, but the process takes time. Your body needs to detoxify, and this doesn't happen overnight. But by switching to natural, plant-based products, you may start to feel better and notice a difference over time.

In nature, there are countless herbs and plants with healing properties. For example, many fruits can help nourish the skin. When you're eating a piece of fruit, try putting a small dab on your face, especially if you're alone and have some time to let it sit. You might be surprised to find that it smooths your skin or reduces fine lines.

These simple, natural solutions can support your body's health and beauty without the risks of harsh chemicals. Nature has powerful, gentle ways of helping us look and feel our best—if we give it the chance!

Prioritizing Health and Awareness

Throughout history, we have been guided by the natural world to nurture and sustain our well-being. In today's complex environment, it's easy to overlook what we expose our bodies to, whether through the food we eat, the products we apply, or the air we breathe. The wisdom of traditional practices and natural remedies reminds us to pause and reconnect with simple, effective ways of caring for ourselves.

Understanding What We Use

Modern products often promise convenience and beauty but may conceal ingredients that are far from beneficial. Reading labels and understanding what goes into everyday items can empower us to make healthier choices. This awareness is a step toward reducing our exposure to potentially harmful substances.

Healing Through Nature

Even after prolonged use of chemical-laden products, the body holds an incredible ability to heal when given the right tools. Plant-based solutions, derived from nature's abundance, offer gentle yet powerful ways to support the body's recovery. These methods may take time but align with the body's natural rhythms to bring about lasting renewal.

Listening to the Body

Our bodies send us signals—through skin reactions, fatigue, or other discomforts—when something is out of balance. Paying attention to these cues and responding with care fosters a deeper relationship with our well-being.

A Holistic Approach

By integrating natural alternatives, eating whole foods, and choosing mindful practices, we honor both ourselves and the environment. As ancient wisdom teaches, what nourishes and sustains us should align with the earth's rhythms, reflecting a harmony that benefits all life.

Choosing natural options and embracing the healing power of plants is more than a personal choice—it's a step toward living in balance with the world around us. Let nature guide your journey toward health and vitality.

Metal Implants: What Are the Risks?

Many people, including family and friends, have metal implants. Some implants work well, but others cause serious problems. Metal implants can release tiny particles of chromium and cobalt into the bloodstream, which can lead to health issues, like cancer and heart problems.

Here are some common concerns with metal implants:

Artificial Hips

Artificial hip implants usually last about 10 to 15 years. However, some metal-on-metal hip implants wear out in just five years. These metal hips can damage the tissue and bone around them. They were meant to be an upgrade from plastic, but they often fail. When they come loose from the bone, they cause more pain and make it difficult for bone cells to grow. If a replacement is needed, it's harder to do the surgery due to the bone loss, and the chances of failure are higher.

Metal Allergies and Pseudotumors

Some people are allergic to the metal in implants, which can cause painful reactions. This reaction may create soft tissue growth around the metal, called a pseudotumor. Sadly, people often don't know they're allergic to the metal until after surgery. If you notice any bad reaction, it's important to tell your doctor quickly, as the metal can affect your bloodstream too.

Knee Implants

Knee implants can also fail if the metal parts become loose. This can lead to:

- Stiffness
- Swelling
- Pain

If the knee pain doesn't go away, it might mean that the body is rejecting the implant. For example, my uncle had a knee implant that caused him a lot of pain. After a long wait, he finally got a new knee replacement, which worked much better for him.

Why Don't Implants Last Longer?

With today's technology, you might expect implants to last at least 20 years. But our bodies aren't made to handle foreign metals and chemicals. Just like prescription drugs, these implants can have harmful effects. Many people experience failures with these implants, which is devastating. They have to go through another painful surgery to remove and replace the implant, hoping it will work better the next time.

Recalls on Implants

Recently, some manufacturers have recalled faulty implants due to complaints from people suffering from the implants' failures. Thankfully, more people are speaking up, and their concerns are finally being heard.

Metal implants can help some people, but for many others, the risks and side effects are serious. If you or someone you know is considering a metal implant, it's important to weigh these risks carefully.

Natural Alternatives to Metal Implants and Herbal Remedies

Metal implants can sometimes cause problems in the body, like inflammation, pain, and allergies. But did you know that there are natural alternatives to metal implants? For those who already have metal implants, there are also herbal and natural remedies that may help reduce some of the side effects.

Natural Alternatives to Metal Implants

If you need a joint replacement or similar surgery, here are some natural options that might help avoid the use of metal:

- Stem Cell Therap
  - Stem cells are cells in the body that can turn into different types of tissues, like bone or cartilage. Doctors can inject these cells into joints to help repair damaged areas, especially in knees and hips. This can sometimes delay or even prevent the need for metal implants.

- Physical Therapy and Exercis
  - Exercise helps strengthen the muscles around joints, which can relieve pain and improve movement. Physical therapy can also teach you safe ways to move, which may help reduce joint stress and delay the need for surgery.

- Herbal Supplements for Joint Health
  - Certain herbal supplements are known to support joint health and reduce pain:
    - Turmeric
      - Known for its anti-inflammatory properties, turmeric can help reduce joint pain.
    - Ginger
      - Ginger is another anti-inflammatory herb that may help with pain relief.
    - Boswellia
      - Also called "Indian frankincense," Boswellia has been used for centuries to reduce inflammation and support joint health.
    - Acupuncture

- Acupuncture is an ancient practice that uses small needles placed in specific points on the body to relieve pain. Studies have shown that acupuncture can help relieve joint pain and may be an alternative to surgery.
- Bone Grafts
  - Bone grafts use natural bone from another part of the body or from a donor to repair damaged bones. This is often used instead of metal in some cases and is especially helpful in dental and certain joint surgeries.

Remedies for Reducing Side Effects of Metal Implants

If you already have a metal implant, here are some natural remedies and tips to support your body and reduce the potential side effects:

- Detoxifying Foods and Herbs
  - Some foods and herbs may help your body detox from any metals that might be released into your bloodstream.

    - Cilantro
      - Known to help remove heavy metals from the body, cilantro can be added to salads or smoothies.
    - Chlorella
      - A type of green algae, chlorella is believed to bind to heavy metals and remove them from the body.
    - Garlic
      - Garlic is rich in antioxidants and may support the liver in filtering out toxins.
    - Anti-Inflammatory Diet
      - Eating foods that reduce inflammation can help lessen the pain and swelling often associated with metal implants. Foods to include:
        - Leafy greens (like spinach and kale)
        - Berries (like blueberries and strawberries)
        - Nuts and seeds (like almonds and chia seeds)

> ▪ Healthy fats (like olive oil and avocados)

Herbal Remedies for Pain and Inflammation

There are herbs that may help relieve pain and swelling around implants:

- Turmeric
  - o This herb has strong anti-inflammatory properties and can be taken as a supplement or added to food.
- Willow Bark
  - o Known as "nature's aspirin," willow bark may help relieve pain naturally.
- Ginger
  - o Ginger not only helps with inflammation but also supports digestion, which can be helpful if you take medications.
- Regular Exercise and Stretching
  - o Gentle exercise and stretching can help keep the muscles around your implant strong, which can help support the area and reduce pain. Low-impact exercises like swimming, walking, or gentle yoga are especially good for joint health.
- Hydration and Proper Nutrition
  - o Drinking plenty of water and eating a balanced diet can help your body flush out any toxins. Water supports kidney function, which plays an important role in removing unwanted substances from the body.

- Massage Therapy
  - o Massage therapy can help relieve tension and improve blood flow around the implant area. This can reduce swelling and help with pain, especially if the implant has caused muscle tightness or discomfort.

Things to Remember

Before trying any natural or herbal remedies, it's always best to talk to your doctor. They can help make sure the remedies are safe for your specific situation, especially if you already have an implant.

Remedies for Hangovers

Have you ever had such a wild night of drinking that you woke up not knowing how you got home, where your keys are, why your knees hurt, or why you're in pajamas? And then, as you try to figure it out, you're hit with a pounding headache, an upset stomach, and other hangover symptoms. So, what can help with a hangover once the fun is over?

Let's start by understanding what causes hangovers. When alcohol is broken down by your liver, it creates a toxic substance called acetaldehyde. This happens more with cheaper wines or spirits, which can be harder on your liver.

Alcohols That Can Cause Stronger Hangovers

To avoid strong hangovers, try to stay away from these drinks:

- Whiskey
- Cheap red wines
- Fruit brandy
- Dark spirits

Instead, go for clear spirits or high-quality red wines that don't contain added sulfites. Organic options are usually better for your liver.

How the Body Processes Alcohol

The liver breaks down alcohol in two phases:

- First Phase
  - Alcohol is turned into less harmful substances with the help of enzymes. This process can create free radicals, which antioxidants help to neutralize. But if you drink too much, it can overwhelm your liver.

- Second Phase
  - The liver makes the toxins from Phase One water-soluble so they can leave your body. If your liver is healthy, it can get rid of these toxins faster. Some herbs can help support and strengthen your liver.

Herbs and Natural Remedies for Hangovers

Here are some natural remedies that may help ease hangover symptoms:

- Ginger

- o Known for reducing nausea and settling an upset stomach. It also helps your metabolism, which can improve detoxification.
- Turmeric
  - o Helps repair liver cells and reduces inflammation and pain.
- Chlorella
  - o A type of algae that supports liver cell repair, removes pollutants from the body, and helps detoxify.
- Mint
  - o Mint helps with digestion and can boost energy, ease nausea, and improve mental clarity.
- Fennel
  - o Great for easing nausea and indigestion. Try making fennel tea to start feeling better.
- Chamomile
  - o Chamomile tea is calming, helps with headaches, and soothes the stomach.
- Parsley
  - o Rich in minerals and chlorophyll, parsley helps remove harmful acids from the body.

Menudo: The Hangover Soup

If you want a hearty meal to help with your hangover, try menudo. This Mexican soup is a popular remedy with lots of spices. You can add onions, cilantro, and even cabbage. Eat it with hot corn tortillas, and by the end of the meal, you might feel a lot better.

Bonus Tip

Some people find that taking one Tylenol before they start drinking can help prevent a hangover. But remember, everyone's metabolism is different, so it might not work for everyone.

These herbs and remedies can help ease hangover symptoms and make you feel better faster.

How to Stop Smoking – No Joking!

Do you know people who smoke? Or have you ever kissed someone who does? It's like kissing an ashtray! Every year, many smokers say, "I'm going to quit one day." But for most, that day never seems to come.

Sometimes friends will show smokers how much money they could save if they stopped buying cigarettes. It's a lot! People with habits like smoking often spend money without thinking about how it adds up.

When I worked at a gas station years ago, some people would ask if they could buy just a couple of cigarettes because they couldn't afford a whole pack but needed their "fix" for the day. I even tried a cigarette once, but I didn't see the appeal. Some people say smoking helps them relax, while others say it keeps them from feeling hungry.

I remember a time when a coworker begged me to trade breaks because she was desperate for a smoke. When I said no, she got really angry and started cursing. If I had known about natural ways to help quit smoking back then, I would have told her about them!

If you or someone you know is trying to quit, here are some herbs that might help:

Herbs That May Help You Quit Smoking

- Skullcap
    - Skullcap can help with withdrawal by calming the body, relaxing the mind, and easing anxiety and depression.
- St. John's Wort
    - St. John's Wort is known to ease withdrawal symptoms, especially for people quitting smoking. It calms the nervous system and can be taken as a tincture (a liquid extract).
- Osha
    - Osha is an herb that helps reduce nicotine cravings. Chewing the root can ease the need for a cigarette.
- Parrot's Beak
    - Parrot's Beak can help people quit smoking by reducing stress and anxiety. It keeps you feeling calm and relaxed, which can make the withdrawal process easier.

Note: If you're pregnant or breastfeeding, wait until after you finish breastfeeding to try these herbs, as we don't know how they might affect babies.

These are just a few natural remedies that may help you quit smoking. If I find more, I'll share them!

If you're reading this and still deciding whether to quit, please remember to think of those around you when you smoke. Some people have trouble breathing around cigarette smoke. Also, please don't throw cigarette butts out of car windows or on sidewalks—let's keep our environment clean.

Thank you for being considerate, and best of luck if you're ready to quit.

Returning to Natural Balance and Supporting Wellness

The human body, as ancient wisdom reminds us, thrives when it aligns with nature's rhythms. Challenges like chronic pain, modern habits, and even the effects of aging often push us to seek solutions. Across generations, original cultures have emphasized the healing power of plants and a lifestyle rooted in balance. These lessons remain profoundly relevant today.

Healing and Alternatives

Modern interventions, whether surgical or chemical, serve valuable purposes, particularly in urgent or severe cases. Yet, integrating natural approaches—be it through mindful nutrition, plant-based remedies, or physical therapies—can support long-term well-being. These methods aim not only to address symptoms but to nurture the body's inherent capacity to heal and adapt.

Cleansing and Detoxification

In a world increasingly dominated by synthetic influences, traditional practices remind us of the value of cleansing the body. Foods, herbs, and rituals that help detoxify can bring clarity and vitality, addressing imbalances caused by modern life.

Mindful Transitions

For those working to overcome dependencies or recover from physical challenges, the journey requires patience and resilience. Herbal allies, emotional support, and mindfulness can serve as guides through these transitions, offering strength and stability.

Harmonious Living

Ultimately, the choices we make—whether to embrace modern innovations, ancient remedies, or both—should reflect our unique needs and values. By listening to our bodies and respecting the wisdom of nature, we create space for healing that respects the interconnectedness of life.

May the lessons of the past and the insights of the present inspire you to pursue health with courage, balance, and gratitude for the earth's gifts.

3 NATURAL ALTERNATIVES TO MEDS

When I first started learning about natural remedies, I was amazed at how many solutions came straight from nature. Herbs, plants, and natural minerals have been used for thousands of years to heal and support the body. Our ancestors relied on these remedies to address everything from minor aches to serious illnesses, often with incredible results. They understood something we've started to forget: the body has an amazing ability to heal itself when it's given the right tools.

Today, we live in a world where prescription drugs are often the first answer to health problems. Don't get me wrong—modern medicine has its place. Prescription drugs can save lives, especially in emergencies or when we need fast relief. But too often, we rely on them as the only solution. What if we could pair the advances of modern medicine with the timeless wisdom of natural remedies? What if we could explore a gentler, more holistic way to heal that works with the body, not against it?

One of the most fascinating things I've learned is how herbs and plants address not just symptoms but the root causes of illness. They work to bring the body back into balance, supporting natural processes rather than overpowering them. While prescription drugs are designed to target specific problems, they often come with side effects that can leave us feeling worse in other ways. Herbs, on the other hand, tend to work more gently, giving the body time to heal fully.

But that doesn't mean we have to choose one over the other. For some, prescription medications are necessary, and that's okay. The key is knowing when to use them and when to explore alternatives. By combining the strengths of modern medicine with the healing power of nature, we can create a balanced approach to health that feels more personal and sustainable.

Prescription Medications or Herbals?

Herbs are plants and natural substances that help bring balance to the body and relieve sickness. Did you know that about 40% of prescription drugs come from plants? But there is a difference in how herbs and prescription drugs work.

How Prescription Drugs Work

Most prescription drugs are created to do one specific thing, focusing on one problem. This concentrated, single-purpose action often makes the drug harder for the body to handle. While these drugs may work quickly, they can also cause side effects that might feel worse than the original symptom.

How Herbs Work

Herbs and plants have been used for centuries to keep people healthy. They are all-natural, and the body tends to respond better to them. Unlike prescription drugs, herbs often work by bringing the body back into balance and targeting the root cause of an illness, not just covering up symptoms.

When we feel sick, it's easy to reach for a quick fix. But while prescription drugs can help fast, they don't always solve the real problem. Herbs, on the other hand, work slowly but can offer lasting healing.

The Best Use for Each

Both prescription drugs and herbs have their place. Prescription medications are very helpful when you need fast results or in emergencies. They have saved many lives! But for chronic conditions that haven't improved with drugs, herbs may be a good alternative.

Herbs, plants, flowers, and minerals are natural healers. They don't work instantly, but over time, they may heal you completely by addressing the source of the problem.

Getting Help from a Herbalist

If you want to use herbs for healing, it's best to go to a licensed herbalist. Herbalists are trained and know exactly what herbs to use, how much to use, and how to find the right mix for each person. They are like doctors for natural healing, helping to find the exact herbs that will work best for you.

Many people today are turning back to natural herbs because they feel that "prescription drugs have too many side effects." A skilled herbalist is essential—they carefully blend the right herbs, like a chemist, to find the perfect dose for each individual. Unlike synthetic drugs, herbs work in harmony with our bodies, which may lead to fewer side effects and more lasting results.

Whether you choose prescription medications, herbal treatments, or a mix of both, remember that each has its benefits. But for lasting health, herbs can be a gentle, natural way to support the body and address the root of many health issues.

Changing Your Quality of Life

Have you ever gone to the pharmacy to buy something for a cold, pain relief, or stomachache? You end up reading all the labels, trying to find something that matches your symptoms, and it feels like you'd have to buy half the shelf to cover everything you need!

It's frustrating, right? And sometimes, you can't even find what you're looking for, which is even worse.

What's Really in Our Medicine?

Have you ever wondered what's actually in the medications we buy? Some of those ingredients have strange, long names. I once bought an aloe gel that claimed to soothe and cool sunburns. But when I read the ingredients, I found that aloe was barely in it! The rest of the bottle was filled with chemicals.

Some of these chemicals, if used for too long, can actually dry out your skin, cause rashes, wrinkles, and even cancer. But they don't tell you that on the bottle. To find out, you'd have to research each ingredient, which most of us don't have time for.

Where Did Our Quality Go?

With today's technology, we're led to believe that our quality of life is better than ever. But why, then, are we seeing more obesity and more sickness?

Our food has changed. It's often over-processed, made to grow faster, and filled with additives. Animals are fed steroids to grow faster and bigger, which means we're eating those things too without realizing it.

Are we blindly accepting all of this?

Time to Open Our Eyes

It's time to open our eyes and start making healthier choices. This affects our lives and the lives of our children. We're allowing chemicals to be put into our food, sometimes even labeled as "healthy" or "organic." But how healthy can it really be if it's filled with hidden chemicals?

What Can We Do?

As consumers, we have the power to make a change. We can start by paying attention to what we buy, reading labels, and choosing natural options when possible. If enough of us start making better choices, companies may start listening.

Let's work together to make sure our food, medicines, and other products are truly safe and healthy for us and for future generations.

Rediscovering Balance Through Nature and Knowledge

In the wisdom carried forward by ancient traditions, the understanding of health is rooted in harmony—between the body, the earth, and the elements that sustain life. The choices we make about how to care for ourselves reflect this balance, whether through modern advancements or the gifts of nature.

The Two Paths of Healing

Both nature's remedies and modern innovations hold unique strengths. While one offers the precision of rapid relief, the other provides a nurturing approach to restoring balance. Choosing between them—or combining their benefits—is not about opposing philosophies but finding what serves the deeper needs of the body and soul.

The Essence of Nature's Remedies

Herbs, plants, and minerals remind us of a time when healing was intertwined with the earth's cycles. These remedies aim not only to relieve symptoms but to address root causes, restoring the natural flow of energy and wellness. Their gentle, slow approach mirrors the patience of the seasons, offering healing that endures.

Modern Tools in a Fast-Paced World

Prescription medications have their place, particularly in emergencies and situations that demand immediate intervention. Their focused design is a testament to human ingenuity, though it reminds us of the importance of mindful use, as quick solutions may sometimes leave deeper imbalances unaddressed.

The Power of Choice

As stewards of our well-being, the power lies in our choices—reading labels, seeking knowledge, and understanding what we put into our bodies. Whether we turn to modern tools or ancestral wisdom, what matters is our commitment to health and to making informed, conscious decisions.

Returning to Intentional Living

By aligning with natural cycles, we embrace a life of awareness. When we choose foods, medicines, and practices that honor the earth and our bodies, we invest in a future where balance is not a luxury but a way of life.

May the wisdom of both paths guide you toward health, harmony, and the empowerment to live fully in the present moment.

Honey, Lemon, and Ginger Tea

Winter is here, and so is flu season! How can we protect ourselves from getting sick?

The most important thing is to wash your hands often and try not to touch your face. It may sound simple, but it really helps. When around other people, keep your mouth closed, and remember, wearing a mask can prevent germs from entering through your nose or mouth.

If you're out on the road and don't have water or hand sanitizer, even baby wipes can help clean your hands. Staying healthy also means getting plenty of rest and eating foods that support your immune system. You don't need a special diet, but adding certain foods can make a difference.

If you feel a cold coming on, try drinking a small glass of wine (just a little!) to help warm you up. Also, keep your home warm, but not too hot.

My mom used to say, "If you keep the house too hot and then go outside, you'll get sick!" I'm not sure if that's true, but everyone has their own way of staying healthy.

How to Make Honey, Lemon, and Ginger Tea

Here's a simple recipe I use to help boost immunity and soothe sore throats:

1. Take 2 lemons – zest them first, then slice them thin.
2. Peel and thinly slice 1 ginger root.
3. In a glass jar, place the lemon slices and ginger. Press down a bit to release the juices.
4. Add the lemon zest, then pour raw honey over everything until the lemon and ginger are fully covered.
5. Close the jar tightly and store it in the refrigerator.

This mixture is delicious in tea, and if you get a sore throat, you can take a spoonful for relief. It's also great for helping you relax and sleep!

How This Tea Helps My Grandson

My grandson, who's seven, has so much energy that he once jumped on our mini trampoline for two hours straight while we watched a movie! I wish I could bottle that energy! When he visits, I make him honey, lemon, and ginger tea. After drinking it, he often feels tired and ready for bed—no more endless bouncing!

Now, every time he visits, he asks for "honey and tea." It's sweet and tasty for him, but for me, it's a great way to keep him healthy. The tea helps him rest, soothes his throat if it's sore, and best of all, it's all natural!

Longer Lashes and Hair with Herbs

I used to have a friend with naturally long, curly eyelashes. She would actually trim them because they were too long and bothered her—she didn't like them! She was so lucky and didn't even realize it.

Many people today spend a lot of money to get thick, beautiful eyelashes. They say the eyes are the windows to the soul, and long lashes are like lovely curtains for those windows. I would love to have thicker, longer lashes, too. I've tried false lashes, and they looked great, but they're expensive and don't last long.

Short lashes can be caused by things like rubbing your eyes a lot. This can pull out lashes or break them, making them shorter. I know I'm guilty of rubbing my eyes often, even when I have false lashes on!

Before you try any remedies to grow your eyelashes, talk to your eye doctor to make sure it's safe for you.

Stress and Hair Growth

Stress can also affect hair growth. When you're stressed, blood flow goes to areas that need it most, which sometimes means less blood flow to your hair and lashes. If possible, try to reduce stress to help your hair grow.

Herbs for Lash and Hair Growth

Here are a few natural remedies that may help grow both eyelashes and hair:

- Rosemary and Cinnamon
  - I've used rosemary and cinnamon for my hair for years, and it really works! Here's how to make a hair growth formula:

    - Boil water in a pot, add 4 cinnamon sticks, and let simmer for 15 minutes.
    - Add 4 sprigs of fresh rosemary and simmer for another 20 minutes, then let it cool.
    - Remove the cinnamon sticks and rosemary, and pour the mixture into a container.

    You can store this in a cool place and use it as a spray to spritz your hair instead of plain water.

- Green Tea
  - Green tea is not only a popular drink but also great for hair health. It helps reduce stress, which can support hair growth.

- Nettle Leaf
  - Nettle leaf is full of collagen and minerals that help promote hair growth. It supports not only the hair on your head but can also be used for lashes and eyebrows.

There are many other herbs that can reduce stress and support hair growth. You just have to find the ones that work best for you.

Natural Breast Enlargement

I remember when I was in junior high and hadn't developed yet. I was tall and skinny, while other girls my age already had breasts. I hadn't hit puberty, and it wasn't until eighth grade that I finally started developing. For me, like many girls, it felt like a big milestone, a sign of growing up—kind of like how young boys wait to get stronger and more muscular.

As we get older, we go through many changes. Some happen naturally, and others come from wanting to look a certain way or feeling pressure to change. Sometimes, even partners or friends make comments about looking more attractive with a different shape, which can be hard to ignore.

If you're interested in trying natural ways to enhance your breasts, there are some herbs that may help. But be careful, as some herbs can affect your hormones. It's always best to talk to a knowledgeable herbalist who can guide you to the safest options.

Herbs for Natural Breast Enhancement

Here are some popular herbs believed to help with breast enhancement:

- Fenugreek
  - Fenugreek seeds are known for their ability to support breast tissue growth. You can soak the seeds in water until they sprout, then eat the sprouts regularly to see changes.
- Flaxseed and Fennel Seeds
  - Both flaxseed and fennel seeds contain compounds that can support breast tissue tone and growth. Adding these seeds to your diet may help over time.
- Wild Yam
  - Wild yam contains plant estrogens that may promote tissue growth by helping the body retain fluid, which gives a fuller look to curves. This is often seen as a bonus benefit.

How Natural Growth Works

The size of a woman's breasts is often determined during puberty. If puberty ends early, some women may remain smaller-chested into adulthood. However, adding certain estrogen-rich foods and herbs to your diet may support natural enhancement.

But keep in mind, the body can only handle so much estrogen. Overdoing it can lead to side effects, so it's important to stay within a healthy limit.

By adding these herbs and foods to your diet safely, you might see natural, subtle changes—no surgery needed!

How to Reduce Breast Size

I've always felt happy with the way I am, but sometimes our bodies don't stop growing in time, and breasts can become larger than we want. Instead of being something to feel good about, they can start to feel heavy and even cause back pain.

I once knew a woman who had surgery to reduce her breast size because of the pain. She said it was like carrying two 20-pound weights on her chest! After surgery, she felt much better. But if you want to try reducing breast size naturally, here are some tips that may help:

Diet Changes for Reducing Breast Size

- Flaxseed and Salmon
    - Eating flaxseed along with salmon (which is high in omega-3s) can help reduce excess fats in the body. Omega-3s are good for burning fat.
- Eat to Feel Full and Lose Weight
    - Choose foods that keep you full but help with healthy weight loss, like chicken, nuts, and vegetables. These foods can support fat loss all over, including in the breasts.
- Limit Dairy
    - Milk and soy milk have high levels of estrogen, which can promote breast growth. Cutting back on dairy can help with breast reduction.
- Add Certain Vegetables
    - Vegetables like kale, cauliflower, broccoli, and cabbage help your body process and reduce extra estrogen, which may help shrink breast tissue.

Herbs and Foods That Support Breast Reduction

- Green Tea
  - Green tea is full of antioxidants and helps boost metabolism, which can help burn calories and fat. Try drinking green tea throughout the day for more energy.
- Ginger Tea
  - Ginger tea is another great option if you get tired of green tea. It helps boost energy, and it's known to support metabolism too.
- Citrus Fruits
  - Oranges, lemons, and limes contain a compound called d-limonene that helps reduce excess estrogen. Adding these fruits to your diet can be helpful.

- Exercise Tips
  - Exercise is also important for reducing body fat, including breast size. If you have larger breasts, you may want to bind or support them well to avoid pain while working out. Always check with your doctor before starting any intense workout.

Final Thoughts

Before trying herbs to lower estrogen, talk to a qualified herbalist to make sure it's safe for you. Different things work for different people, so it's important to find the right approach for your body.

Consider trying these natural methods before thinking about surgery. Always remember to do what feels right for you!

Leg Nerve Pain

Many people today wake up with pain in their legs or feet. For some, the pain comes and goes, while for others, it never seems to stop.

Living with constant leg pain is tough, especially when you're trying to stay active. Telling your doctor may lead to more prescription drugs, which often come with side effects. You might wonder if there's anything else you can try.

One natural remedy that might help is apple cider vinegar. It's been around for centuries and is commonly found in homes. Apple cider vinegar has minerals like potassium, magnesium, and calcium. Because it's a natural anti-inflammatory, it can help reduce swelling in painful areas.

How to Use Apple Cider Vinegar for Nerve Pain

Take 2 or 3 tablespoons of apple cider vinegar, mix it with warm water, and drink it. Some people find relief from their pain after using it regularly.

Common Causes of Nerve Pain (Neuropathy)

Neuropathy, or nerve pain, can be caused by:

- Diabetes
- Infections
- Traumatic injuries
- Alcoholism

Types of Nerve Damage

There are three types of nerves that can be affected by neuropathy:

- Motor Nerves
  - Motor nerves control our movements. When these nerves are damaged, it becomes hard to move, and muscles can feel stiff or weak. You may experience muscle spasms or twitching.
- Sensory Nerves
  - Sensory nerves send messages to the brain, like when you feel something hot or cold. With sensory nerve damage, you may lose the ability to feel temperature changes, experience numbness, tingling, or lose coordination.
- Autonomic Nerves
  - Autonomic nerves control things like bladder function, blood pressure, sweating, heart rate, and breathing. Damage to these nerves can affect basic body functions.

How to Manage Neuropathy and Leg Pain

Prioritize Tasks

Try to spread out your activities so you don't overdo it. For example, do your grocery shopping on one day and other errands on another. This way, your body has time to rest.

Take Breaks and Stay Active

It's okay to take breaks when you go for walks, mow the lawn, or work in the garden. These activities are good for you because they keep you moving, but remember not to push yourself too hard.

Ask for Help When Needed

Sometimes, it's hard to ask for help because we want to stay independent. But asking for help shows wisdom. It means you know your limits, and that's smart.

Get Enough Rest and Stay Positive

Make sure to get plenty of sleep, and try to stay positive. Keep moving forward, one day at a time.

With the right balance of rest, activity, and some natural remedies, you may find some relief from leg nerve pain. Remember to listen to your body and do what feels best for you.

Lesson Learned from Jack's Heart Attack

I want to tell you a true story about my friend Jack. He's tall, slender, and very active. Jack loves fishing, camping, hunting, and archery, and he's always out enjoying nature. His doctor told him to exercise, eat healthy, and take his medication, so he followed all the instructions. But one day, Jack had a third heart attack.

I rushed to the hospital as soon as I heard. When I got there, Jack was lying in bed with nurses checking his vitals and doctors coming in and out. They looked at him but didn't say much. Then, one of the nurses came in, looked at his chart, and said, "That's the problem!"

I asked her what she meant. She told us Jack's body was low on potassium and magnesium. These two minerals are very important for the heart, like a spark plug that keeps it going. As we age, our bodies need more of them to keep the heart healthy.

While I sat there waiting for hours, not knowing if Jack would be okay, not a single doctor mentioned potassium or magnesium. I once had a heart attack myself and was never told about these minerals either. Why keep this a secret? If we know about this, we might help prevent more heart problems.

After recovering, Jack started taking potassium and magnesium along with his vitamins, and he's been doing great ever since. He's back to being active and even joins us for archery competitions where he loves to show off his skills.

If you ever wake up with painful leg cramps, potassium and magnesium can help with that too. As we get older, our bodies don't work as they used to, so we need a little extra help to stay in balance.

Remember to keep seeing your doctor and always ask questions about your health. Our bodies sometimes give us hints when something is wrong. If we listen closely, we might catch these signals before bigger problems happen. Stay safe and take care of your heart.

Listening to the Signals of the Heart and Body

In the wisdom passed down by ancestral traditions, the heart is seen as not just a physical organ, but as a center of vitality and connection to life. When it faces challenges, it reminds us to honor the balance of body, spirit, and the gifts of the Earth that sustain us.

The Power of Awareness

The body often speaks in whispers before it shouts. Subtle signs, like fatigue or discomfort, may signal the need for deeper care and attention. Just as an eagle watches the land from above, we too must be watchful of the signals our bodies send, responding with mindfulness and care.

Nourishment from Nature

The Earth provides an abundance of what the heart needs to remain strong. Essential minerals and nutrients are among these gifts, nurturing our internal rhythms and ensuring balance. By understanding and integrating these into our daily lives, we align with the natural cycles that promote wellness.

The Strength of Inquiry and Vigilance

One lesson is clear: it is vital to ask questions and seek knowledge about our health. Like the elders who share stories to guide and protect, listening to experts while staying curious ensures we are active participants in our well-being.

Restoration Through Balance

Maintaining heart health is a reflection of balance in all aspects of life. It involves movement to keep the body strong, rest to allow for renewal, and a connection to both the physical and emotional needs that sustain us.

Gratitude and Care

When challenges come, they also bring opportunities to deepen our understanding and appreciation of life. By nurturing the heart—physically and emotionally—we cultivate resilience and the ability to thrive.

Let us honor the lessons learned and take them to heart, knowing that the body and spirit thrive when treated with care, curiosity, and respect for the gifts that nature provides.

Erectile Dysfunction

Erectile Dysfunction, or ED, is a problem that affects a lot of men, but most don't like to talk about it. It feels embarrassing for some, and they may worry about letting down their partner or fear that others will find out. But ED is more common than you might think, and it's nothing to be ashamed of.

Why Does ED Happen?

There are many reasons why ED can happen. Sometimes, the cause is physical, like poor blood flow, stress, or lack of sleep. Other times, it's a mix of things, including emotional stress or changes in health. As we get older, our bodies may need a little extra care to keep everything working well. ED can be a signal that your body needs more rest, better nutrition, or a healthier lifestyle.

In some cases, ED can also point to more serious health issues like heart disease or prostate problems. That's why it's important not to ignore it. If ED is bothering you, don't give up! There are natural ways to help that don't involve prescription drugs, and making small changes can make a big difference.

Steps to Help Improve Erectile Dysfunction Naturally

- Eat Right and Stay Active
  - One of the best ways to help with ED is by eating healthy foods and staying active. Eating well and getting exercise can improve blood flow, which is key to helping with ED. Over time, making these healthy choices can give your body the energy and strength it needs.

    Remember, you're not the same as when you were 20, but that doesn't mean you can't stay active and fit. The right food and exercise can help you feel better, look better, and keep your body working well.

- Try Adding Certain Fruits to Your Diet
  - Some fruits are especially helpful when it comes to blood flow, which is important for improving ED. Fruits like bananas, watermelon, and papayas contain a lot of potassium, which helps keep blood vessels open and blood flowing smoothly. Better blood flow to the whole body, including the penis, can help reduce ED.

    Try having these fruits as snacks or adding them to your meals. Not only are they tasty, but they also provide important nutrients that support heart health and circulation.

- Keep Your Veins and Arteries Healthy
  - Healthy veins and arteries are essential for good blood flow. By eating right and exercising, you help keep your blood vessels clean and open, allowing blood to flow more easily. This not only supports healthy blood pressure and heart health, but it also helps improve ED by making sure blood can reach where it needs to go.

    Certain foods and drinks can clog your arteries, making it harder for blood to flow freely. Avoid foods high in unhealthy fats, like fried or processed foods, and try to drink plenty of water. Good hydration also supports blood flow and keeps your body running smoothly.

- Stay Positive and Reduce Stress
  - A positive mindset can make a huge difference. Worry and stress can make ED worse, so it's helpful to focus on relaxing and staying optimistic. If you feel worried about ED, remember that there are solutions, and you're not alone. Think about past happy moments and try to relax. Having a

positive attitude and practicing relaxation can help lower stress, which benefits the whole body, including your ability to perform well.

- Get Enough Rest
    - o Sleep is one of the best things you can do for your health. Getting enough rest gives your body a chance to recover, balance hormones, and restore energy. Sleep is especially important for men, as lack of sleep can decrease testosterone levels and increase stress, both of which can make ED worse.

Making small, healthy changes can help reduce or even reverse ED. Remember, it's important to care for your body with good food, exercise, hydration, rest, and a positive attitude. These changes may not work overnight, but with time, you can feel stronger and more confident. It's a natural way to feel more like yourself again, and it's worth the effort to improve your health and quality of life.

Honoring the Balance of Wellness and Vitality

In the traditions of the ancient Americas, the harmony of body, mind, and spirit is seen as essential for vitality and well-being. When challenges arise, such as those affecting physical strength or energy, they are viewed as invitations to reconnect with the rhythms of nature and restore balance within ourselves.

Listening to the Signals of the Body

The body speaks in subtle ways, and challenges are often reminders to care for its needs. Issues related to energy or circulation reflect a need to strengthen life's flow—through nourishment, movement, rest, and peace of mind. The wisdom of our ancestors teaches that when the roots of a tree are nourished, the branches grow strong. Likewise, when we tend to the foundation of our health, vitality returns naturally.

The Power of Natural Remedies and Lifestyle

The Earth provides all we need to heal and thrive. Certain foods and herbs have long been used to support energy, circulation, and endurance. Combined with gentle movement, deep rest, and joyful living, these gifts of nature help restore balance.

By embracing nourishing foods, moving with purpose, and breathing deeply, the body's strength and spirit's vitality are renewed. Each step toward balance supports the whole being.

Strength in the Heart and Mind

Emotional peace is as important as physical health. Worry and stress can cloud the mind, but when we calm the spirit and trust the body's ability to heal, we discover our natural strength. Gratitude, mindfulness, and connection to those we love can lift the spirit, allowing renewal and vitality to flow freely.

Patience and Respect for the Process

Healing is a journey, not a race. The lessons of the Earth remind us that all growth takes time, like a seed that slowly becomes a towering tree. With patience, commitment, and a gentle approach, the path forward becomes clear, and vitality returns in its own rhythm.

Through honoring the wisdom of balance and nurturing the sacred connection between body and spirit, we are reminded of the incredible potential for renewal that exists within each of us. This is the way of resilience and strength, rooted in the rhythms of nature and the enduring spirit of life.

What Are the Benefits of Fasting?

You might have heard someone say, "I'm fasting," when they turn down food. It might make you wonder: Is fasting good for the body? Can skipping meals actually be healthy? Let's look at what fasting is and some of the surprising ways it can help your body and mind.

What Is Fasting?

Fasting means not eating for a certain period of time. There are different ways to fast:

- Intermittent Fasting
  - You fast for certain hours in the day, like skipping breakfast and only eating between noon and 8 p.m.
- Alternate-Day Fasting
  - You eat normally one day and fast the next.
- Full-Day Fasting

o   You fast for a full 24 hours, usually only drinking water or tea.

People fast for different reasons. Some do it to lose weight, while others do it for health, focus, or even spiritual reasons. Fasting has been around for centuries, but today, more people are discovering its health benefits.

Benefits of Fasting

Helps with Weight Loss

Fasting can be a good way to lose weight, especially with intermittent fasting. When you fast, you eat less food overall, and your body starts to burn fat for energy. This helps lower blood sugar and can even improve your metabolism (how your body burns calories).

Tip: After fasting, don't overeat or binge on junk food. Try eating balanced meals with fruits, vegetables, and protein to make the most of the benefits.

Makes You Enjoy Food More

Fasting can make you appreciate food more. When you take the time to chew and enjoy each bite, your brain has time to process what you're eating and send signals to your stomach, helping you feel full sooner. When we rush, we tend to eat too much.

Tip: Slow down and savor each bite. This simple trick can help you eat less and feel satisfied, even after smaller portions.

Adjusts to Your Activity Level

If you have a very active job or are always moving, your body will need more fuel. But if your job isn't physically demanding, you may need less food. Fasting helps you become more aware of your eating habits and match them to your activity level.

I learned this myself. When I had an active job, I was always hungry, but when I had to stay home due to an injury, I gained weight because I kept eating the same amount. I learned to adjust my food intake to my activity level, which helped me stay at a healthy weight.

Improves Brain Function and Lowers Inflammation

Fasting doesn't just help the body; it helps the mind too. Fasting can make you think more clearly because it gives the body a break from constantly digesting food. It also helps reduce inflammation, which is the body's way of healing itself but can be harmful if it happens too much. Lower inflammation is good for your heart and can reduce pain in your joints. Studies also show that fasting can lower bad cholesterol, which keeps your heart healthy.

Best of all, fasting may help you live longer by giving your body time to rest, repair, and strengthen itself.

Boosts Energy

At first, fasting might seem like it would make you feel tired, but many people find they actually have more energy while fasting. The body uses stored fat for fuel, which can feel steady and energizing. Fasting also lets the body take a break from working hard on digestion, so it can focus energy elsewhere.

Types of Fasting

Not every type of fasting works for everyone. Here are some options you might consider:

Intermittent Fasting (e.g., fasting for 16 hours and eating only during an 8-hour window)
Alternate-Day Fasting (e.g., eating normally one day and fasting the next)
Water Fasting (drinking only water for a set time)
Partial Fasting (restricting certain foods or meals but not all food)
Each method has its own benefits, so it's important to choose one that feels right. Research the different options and speak to your doctor about what would work best for you, especially if you have any health concerns.

Tips to Make Fasting Easier

Stay Hydrated

Drink plenty of water while fasting to help prevent hunger and keep you feeling full. Herbal teas or lemon water are good options that add flavor without calories.

Find a Fasting Buddy

Fasting can be easier when you have a friend or family member doing it with you. You can encourage each other and share tips to stay on track, especially during difficult moments.

Focus on Your Goal

Remember why you started fasting. Whether it's for weight loss, health, or mental clarity, keeping your goal in mind can help you stay focused.

Start Slowly

If fasting is new to you, try easing into it. Begin with short fasting periods, then gradually increase the time as your body adjusts. This can help prevent feeling overly hungry or tired.

Eat Healthy When Not Fasting

Fasting works best when paired with healthy eating. During your eating window, focus on fruits, vegetables, whole grains, and lean proteins to nourish your body and keep you energized.

Fasting isn't just about skipping meals—it's about giving your body a break and enjoying the benefits. Give it a try and see how it works for you.

The Power of Rest and Renewal: Lessons from Nature

In the wisdom of my ancestors, balance and rhythm are seen as essential to life. Just as the Earth cycles through seasons of growth and dormancy, so too can the human body benefit from periods of rest and renewal. The practice of fasting mirrors these natural rhythms, offering the body a chance to restore, cleanse, and rejuvenate.

Embracing Natural Cycles

Fasting is not a deprivation but a return to simplicity, an alignment with the natural cycles of life. It allows the body to pause from constant activity, much like the way the land rests in winter to prepare for the abundance of spring. This pause can bring clarity to the mind and strength to the body, fostering harmony within.

The Healing Pause

Sacred teachings remind us that healing often requires stillness. By giving the body a break from constant digestion, fasting encourages a shift inward, allowing energy to be redirected toward repair and restoration. This quieting of the physical can open pathways for spiritual and mental clarity, much like a still pond reflects the sky more clearly.

Awareness and Gratitude

Periods of fasting can deepen our appreciation for nourishment, fostering a sense of gratitude for the food we eat and the energy it provides. In many traditions, fasting is also a time for reflection and connection—an opportunity to honor the sacred relationship between the self and the sustenance provided by the Earth.

Balance in Practice

Fasting, like all practices, requires mindfulness. Just as the Earth's rhythms teach us to act with care, fasting should be approached with respect for the body's needs. Whether through gentle pauses or longer periods of rest, the practice should honor individual balance and well-being.

A Lesson from Nature

The ancestors teach us to observe the natural world for guidance. Animals fast instinctively during times of healing or transition, trusting the wisdom of their bodies. By listening to our own inner signals, we can find the rhythm that best supports our health and vitality.

As the elders say, "Rest is the breath of life, and in stillness, strength is born." Fasting, when embraced with care and intention, becomes more than a health practice—it is a way of aligning with the sacred rhythms of existence, nurturing both body and spirit.

Healthy Foods and Herbs to Help Treat Arthritis

Do you remember being a kid, running around, jumping, rolling down hills, riding bikes, or skating? You'd fall, get back up, and do it all over again. Those were fun days that seemed like they'd never end—but they did. What happened? Life happened.

As we grow older, we stop playing as much. These days, we don't go outside unless it's to walk the dog, get the mail, take out the trash, or mow the lawn. Then, technology came along and made things even worse. Now, we move even less.

Lately, things have gotten even harder because many of us have had to stay home. We're stuck inside, looking at our phones more than ever, even when we're with family or friends. It's strange, isn't it? We've stopped paying attention to the world around us.

Meanwhile, the food we eat has changed, too. Big companies are stripping the soil of its nutrients, which makes our food less healthy. Our bodies try their best to keep going, but without enough nutrients, they can't fight off illness and disease as well as they should.

This affects future generations, too. Mothers with poor nutrition give birth to weaker children. Each generation becomes less healthy than the one before. We need to make a change. Growing our own food is a great place to start.

Eating better can even help with conditions like arthritis. Arthritis is a painful disease, and for some people, it's so bad they can't walk or use their hands properly. But the right foods and herbs can help reduce pain and inflammation.

Foods and Herbs That Can Help Arthritis

- Ginger
  - o Ginger is great for arthritis. It helps with joint inflammation and is a tasty addition to meals.

- Green Tea
  - o Green tea is another powerful anti-inflammatory. It's full of antioxidants and can be enjoyed as a drink or added to recipes.

- Turmeric
  - o Turmeric is a flavorful spice with a key ingredient called curcumin. Curcumin has strong anti-inflammatory properties and can be added to many dishes.

- Bananas
  - o Bananas are rich in potassium and magnesium, which can help reduce joint pain.

- Blueberries
  - Blueberries are packed with antioxidants that help protect your body from inflammation.

- Healthy Fats
  - Healthy fats are also important. Foods like salmon, avocado, walnuts, almonds, and olive oil can help your joints and overall health.

- Water
  - Don't forget water! Staying hydrated is crucial for keeping your body healthy.

There are many foods and herbs that can help your body heal itself. Experiment with these options to find the right combination that works best for you. Making these changes can improve your health and reduce arthritis pain.

How to Treat Nail and Foot Fungus Naturally

Do you struggle with embarrassing foot or nail fungus? You're not alone! Many people deal with these issues, but the good news is that there are natural remedies that can help.

Smelly Feet Fix

When I was younger, I had a bad case of smelly feet. Someone told me to try a bleach soak, and it worked!

Here's what to do:

- Mix 1/3 cup of bleach with 2 gallons of warm water.
- Soak your feet for an hour, then rinse.
- Repeat if necessary.

Treating Nail Fungus

Nail fungus is harder to get rid of, but with patience and consistent care, you can treat it.

Start with a Soak

- Fill a tub with water as hot as your feet can handle.

- Add tea tree oil to the water for its antifungal properties.
- Soak your feet until your nails feel soft.
- Trim and Clean

- Once your nails are soft, clean underneath and trim them carefully.

Home Remedies for Nail Fungus

After cleaning and drying your feet, try these remedies:

- Vick's Vapor Rub

    o Apply to the tops of your nails and under them if possible.
    o Use daily until the fungus is gone.
    o Bonus: It can also smooth dry feet and feels refreshing!

- Snake Root Extract

    o This herbal remedy can clear fungus in about three months.
    o Consult a knowledgeable herbalist before use.

- Tea Tree Oil

    o Apply directly to the nail twice daily.
    o Tea tree oil absorbs into the nail to fight the fungus.

- Vinegar Soak

    o Mix equal parts vinegar and warm water.
    o Soak your feet for at least 20 minutes.

- Listerine Soak

    o Soak your feet in Listerine for 20 minutes.
    o Its eucalyptus, thymol, and menthol fight fungus and bacteria.

- Garlic

    o Crush fresh garlic and apply it to your toes.
    o Or take garlic capsules to fight fungus from the inside out.

- Black Tea Soak

       o   Brew a tub of black tea and soak your feet.

- Epsom Salt Soak

     o   Add Epsom salt to warm water and soak your feet.
     o   It's great for fighting nail and foot fungus.

Prevention is Key

The best way to avoid nail fungus is to protect your feet:

Always wear foot coverings at pools, gyms, and hotel showers.

Keep your feet dry and clean.

Fungus is tough to get rid of, but with these tips and some patience, you can heal your nails and keep your feet healthy!

What Can I Do About Chronic Fatigue Syndrome (CFS)?

Do you ever feel so tired that no amount of rest helps? You sleep, try to relax, or even take something to help you rest, but you still wake up feeling just as tired as when you went to bed. It's an endless cycle, and it can feel hopeless.

This condition is called chronic fatigue syndrome (CFS).

Doctors don't fully understand CFS. Some think it might be caused by a virus, stress, or a mix of different factors. The truth is, there's no single known cause, and many illnesses can mimic its symptoms.

There's also no specific test to diagnose CFS, but it most often affects women over 40 or 50. Possible causes include:

- Viral infections
- Hormonal imbalances
- Chronic stress
- Weak immune system

Some researchers think CFS could be the result of multiple infections, especially these three:

- EBV (Epstein-Barr Virus)
- Ross River Virus
- Coxiella burnetii

Don't Lose Hope

Having CFS doesn't mean life is over. When one door closes, another one opens. Even though the journey can be tough, there are ways to manage it and make life better.

One important discovery is how our mitochondria—tiny energy factories inside our cells—work. Mitochondria produce energy in the form of ATP (adenosine triphosphate), which powers our cells and keeps our bodies moving. If mitochondria aren't healthy, your energy levels drop, leading to the extreme fatigue that's common with CFS.

The goal is to protect and strengthen your mitochondria to keep your body functioning.

How to Manage CFS

While there's no cure yet, there are steps you can take to make life easier:

- Identify Energy Drains

  o Pay attention to activities that make you feel more tired.
  o Start by focusing on managing those tasks.

- Pace Yourself

  o Spread out your activities to avoid over-exertion. For example:
  o Shop for clothes one day and groceries another.
  o Do laundry one day and vacuum the next.
  o Taking your time helps prevent extreme fatigue and keeps you moving.

- Accept Good and Bad Days

  o CFS symptoms can come and go. Some days, you'll feel better than others.
  o Do what you can on good days, but don't overdo it.

- Stay Active (When Possible)

- o Even light activity can help keep your body moving and prevent stiffness.
- o Avoid giving in completely on your bad days—small steps matter.

- Stay Positive

  - o It's easy to feel discouraged, but staying hopeful and motivated can make a big difference.

Managing CFS takes time and patience. Scientists are still searching for a cure, but until then, focus on what you can control. Don't give up, and keep smiling—you're stronger than you think!

Poultices: Nature's First Aid

Have you ever gone camping or hiking, set up your tent, and gone for a walk? Everything seems perfect until—slap!—a mosquito bites you. More keep coming, and soon you're heading back to camp. On the way, you trip and scrape your hands and knees on some rocks.

Then you realize… you forgot the first aid kit! But you do have a book about healing plants. Luckily, it shows you how to make a poultice using plants found in the wild.

Plants You Can Use for Poultices

Here are some plants that are great for making poultices:

- Plantain
- Yarrow
- Mullein
- Usnea

You can use one plant or combine several to make a poultice.

Fun fact: Mullein is soft and fluffy, so if you ever forget toilet paper, it's a helpful substitute!

How to Make and Use a Poultice

- Clean the Wound

- o Always clean the wound thoroughly before applying a poultice.

- Prepare the Plant(s)

  - o Crush the fresh plant leaves to release their juices.
  - o If using dry herbs, crush them, add some water to make a paste, and mix well.

- Apply the Poultice

  - o Place the crushed plant or paste directly on the wound.

- Cover and Repeat

  - o Cover the poultice with a clean cloth or bandage to keep it moist.
  - o Change the poultice when it dries out and reapply as needed.

Best Plant Combinations

A mix of plantain and mullein works wonders:

- Plantain
  - o Speeds up healing.

- Mullein
  - o Reduces pain and enhances plantain's effects.

Together, these herbs are a powerhouse for healing wounds and easing discomfort.

Be Prepared

It's always smart to carry an herbal book or an herbal toolbox in your car or backpack. These can come in handy when you least expect it.

Harvesting Herbs the Right Way

When gathering herbs, remember to:

- Be gentle with the plants.

- Only take what you need.
- Avoid uprooting a plant unless you need the root or want to transplant it.
- Clip leaves carefully, leaving enough on the plant for it to keep growing.
- Dry herbs during the summer so you have a supply ready for winter.

Next Time You're Outdoors…

If you forget your first aid kit, don't worry! With your herbal knowledge and a plant guidebook, you can handle unexpected scrapes, bruises, or insect bites. Nature has your back.

Embracing Ancient Wisdom in the Wild

Tribal teachings from my ancestors emphasize that nature provides for all who respect its balance. From the smallest sprout to the towering tree, plants offer their strength, wisdom, and healing when approached with gratitude and care.

The Gifts of the Earth

The ancestors believed that every plant carries a purpose. Some nourish the body, while others heal wounds or protect against harm. In moments of need, nature reveals its remedies to those who take the time to observe, learn, and listen.

The Art of Healing with Plants

Creating remedies from plants is an act of both knowledge and respect. The process of preparing a poultice, for example, mirrors the sacred relationship between humans and the Earth—an exchange of care and life. Using leaves, roots, or flowers for healing reflects a timeless bond and the innate wisdom of the natural world.

Stewardship and Gratitude

The old ways teach us to harvest plants mindfully, taking only what is needed and ensuring the land can replenish itself. This practice honors the spirit of the plant and maintains the balance of the ecosystem, reminding us that we are caretakers, not owners, of the Earth's gifts.

Preparedness and Trust in Nature

The wisdom of the ancestors reminds us that life's challenges, whether a scrape or an unexpected turn, can be met with trust in the Earth's provisions. Carrying knowledge of plants and their uses is like carrying a piece of the forest's resilience, offering peace of mind in uncertain moments.

The Spirit of Connection

Applying a poultice or using a healing herb is more than a practical act; it is a ceremony of connection. Through touch, thought, and intention, we align ourselves with the energy of the natural world, inviting its healing power to flow through us.

As the elders often say, "The Earth has all you need if you walk gently and ask with respect." In every leaf and root lies a story of healing, a reminder of the harmony between humanity and the living world. Let us honor this bond and walk forward with gratitude and care for the gifts nature so freely offers.

Room Temperature or Ice-Cold Water: Does It Matter?

Have you ever been enjoying a tall glass of ice-cold water when someone tells you, "Cold water is bad for you," but they don't explain why?

Let's clear this up: both cold water and room temperature water are good for you because they keep you hydrated, which is the most important thing. But each has its benefits depending on the situation.

Room Temperature Water

Best Time to Drink: After meals or before bed.

Why It's Helpful:

It supports digestion, especially after eating a big meal.
It's gentler on your stomach and easier for your body to absorb.

However, one downside is that room temperature water can make you feel less thirsty, so you might drink less of it, which isn't ideal for staying hydrated.

Cold Water

Best Time to Drink: During or after a workout.

Why It's Helpful:

It cools your body down and gives you an energy boost.
It helps your body produce adrenaline, which can improve your motivation and focus.

Ice-cold water also tends to make you drink more because it's refreshing, which can help you stay better hydrated.

Cold Showers vs. Hot Showers

Now, let's talk about showers. Does it matter if you take a cold or hot one? It turns out, yes!

Cold Showers

At first, the thought of a cold shower might not sound appealing, but they have surprising health benefits:

Improves Blood Circulation: Cold water makes your blood flow faster to keep your internal organs warm.
Boosts Your Immune System: Cold showers increase your metabolic rate, which helps produce more white blood cells to fight illness.
Increases Energy and Mood: The shock of cold water wakes you up, stimulates your body, and releases hormones that can reduce depression. It's like a natural "happiness reset."
Healthier Skin: Cold water doesn't dry out your skin like hot water does. Instead, it helps keep your skin moisturized and healthy.
When to Take a Cold Shower: In the morning. It's a great way to wake up and energize yourself for the day ahead.

Hot Showers

Hot showers feel comforting, but they can dry out your skin, which isn't ideal. They're still great for relaxing your muscles, but overdoing hot showers can strip your skin of natural oils.

The Bottom Line

Both room temperature and cold water have their advantages, and the same goes for showers. Choose based on what your body needs:

For hydration: Drink cold water when you need energy or are working out. Go for room temperature water after meals or before bed.

For showers: Use cold water for a boost in energy, better circulation, and healthier skin. Save hot showers for muscle relaxation, but don't overdo them.

Now you're ready to make smarter choices for your water and shower habits!

Getting into Hot Water

Have you ever come home feeling tired, achy, and just wanting to relax and forget about your day?

I've been there. When I was younger, I'd fill the tub with hot water, climb in, and sometimes even fall asleep. One time, I woke up because my back started to feel cold. I reached for the covers, heard water splashing, and realized I was still in the tub! I promised myself I wouldn't do that again—but I did.

The next time, I made the water as hot as I could stand. At first, it felt amazing, but soon I felt so weak I could barely lift my arms. It felt like my whole body was weighed down. I managed to get out of the tub and into my bed, where I passed out. I woke up the next morning and told myself, never again.

Since then, I've learned that hot showers are a safer way to relax.

The Benefits of Hot Showers

Hot showers are great for relaxing and relieving tension. Here's why:

Relieves Stiff Muscles

Let the hot water run over your stiff shoulders or neck for a few minutes. Gently roll your shoulders or massage your neck as the water melts away tension.

Helps with Congestion

When you're congested from a cold, a hot shower can help you breathe easier.

For extra relief, rub Vicks Vapor Rub on your chest before getting in. Stand in the steam for a few minutes, then get out when you can breathe more easily.

Eases Migraines and Cramps

Hot water expands blood vessels, improving blood flow. This can help with migraines and menstrual cramps, bringing much-needed relief.

Promotes Better Sleep

A hot shower before bed can relax your muscles and help you sleep better.

Alternating Hot and Cold Showers

Did you know switching between hot and cold water in the shower has even more benefits?

Improves Circulation

Cold water makes your blood rush to warm your core. Hot water expands your blood vessels and increases blood flow.

Alternate between 1 minute of cold water and 1 minute of hot water to boost circulation.

Detoxifies Your Body

Improved blood flow helps deliver oxygen and nutrients to your muscles and organs while flushing out toxins.

Cleans and Refreshes Skin

Alternating hot and cold water opens and cleanses your pores, removing trapped dirt and oil. This can lead to healthier skin and may even help reduce acne.

Hot water, whether in a bath or shower, has amazing benefits, but it's important to use it wisely. If you've never tried alternating hot and cold water in your showers, give it a shot—it might leave you feeling more refreshed and energized.

Looking back, I wish I had known about these tips as a teenager. They would've helped me with sore muscles and even acne. But it's never too late to start using the healing power of water to improve your well-being.

Water's Wisdom in Balance and Renewal

The teachings of my ancestors remind us that water is a sacred element, vital to life and a source of both physical and spiritual healing. Tribal teachings from the Americas highlight the adaptability of water, flowing effortlessly to meet the needs of the Earth and its people. Whether cold or warm, still or moving, water offers unique gifts to nurture and restore balance within us.

The Dual Nature of Water

Water's essence lies in its ability to transform and adapt, much like the cycles of life. Cold water invigorates, energizing the body and awakening the senses, while warm water soothes, easing tension and promoting relaxation. Both are gifts, offering what is needed depending on the moment and the individual.

Hydration and Harmony

The ancestors understood the importance of staying connected to the Earth's elements. Drinking water, whether cool or room temperature, is an act of self-care that nourishes the body and sustains life. Choosing the temperature that aligns with your needs reflects the wisdom of listening to your body and honoring its unique rhythm.

The Cleansing Power of Showers

Showers, much like rain, are not just for cleansing the body but for refreshing the spirit. Cold water invigorates, enhancing circulation and awakening the mind. Warm water comforts, relaxing muscles and encouraging stillness. Alternating between the two mirrors the natural ebb and flow of life, fostering renewal and balance.

Healing Through Connection

In cultural traditions, water ceremonies often symbolize purification and renewal. Engaging with water, whether through mindful hydration or intentional bathing, can be a personal ceremony that connects us to nature's healing cycles. This connection nurtures both body and spirit, offering a reminder of water's sacred role in sustaining life.

Lessons from Water

Water teaches us the importance of adaptability and balance:

Flow with the Moment: Cold or warm, water offers what is needed in each situation.

Honor Your Needs: Choose what supports your well-being, just as water shapes itself to the Earth's contours.

Embrace Renewal: Allow water to refresh not just the body but the mind and spirit as well.

As the elders say, "Water carries the song of life; let it sing to your soul." By embracing water in its many forms, we align ourselves with its wisdom, restoring balance, vitality, and peace to our lives.

4 MIND BODY CONNECTION

When I first heard the phrase "mind-body connection," it sounded a bit mysterious, almost like something out of a movie. I wondered, could our thoughts really affect how we feel physically? The more I learned, the more I realized how powerful the connection truly is. Every thought we have—whether positive or negative—can send signals throughout our body, shaping how we experience the world around us. It's like having an invisible bridge between your brain and your body, constantly sending messages back and forth.

I've experienced it myself. Have you ever been so stressed or worried about something that your stomach hurt or your head started pounding? That's your mind influencing your body. On the flip side, think about how your body feels after hearing exciting news or when you're proud of something you've done. You stand taller, breathe easier, and feel full of energy. These moments show how deeply connected our mental and physical states are.

The great news is that this connection isn't just about reacting to life—it's something we can learn to influence and strengthen. By changing the way we think, we can change the way we feel. Positive thoughts can lead to physical healing, better energy, and even a stronger immune system. And the best part? It doesn't require expensive tools or complicated techniques—just a little practice in how we think about ourselves and the world.

Not a Drop of Blood

I've talked before about how powerful our thoughts are. If you believe something to be true, your mind will make it feel real. There's a story about a scientist from Arizona who wanted to prove just how strong the mind can be. He wanted to show that what your mind believes can either heal you or harm you, depending on what you think is true.

The scientist needed someone to take part in his experiment, someone who had nothing to lose. So, he spoke to a man on death row in prison. The scientist told him that instead of dying in the electric chair, it would be easier for him to die by slowly bleeding out. The scientist explained that it would take longer, but the man would fall asleep without pain. "You wouldn't even know you died," the scientist assured him. The man agreed to go along with the plan.

The scientists tied the man to a stretcher, securing his arms and legs so he couldn't move. Then, they made a small cut on his wrist. It wasn't deep enough to kill him, but it was deep enough to bleed and cause some pain. Under the cut, they placed a pan so the man could hear the blood dripping. What he didn't know was that the scientists had set up an IV bag below his wrist. They had timed it to drip slowly, just like blood would.

As time passed, the scientist slowly made the drips slower and quieter. The man couldn't hear the drops like he did earlier. He started to feel weaker and thought that he was losing more and more blood. He looked paler and paler, believing that he was running out of blood.

Then, the scientist turned off the IV bag. The man could no longer hear the sound of blood dripping. He started to panic. He had trouble breathing and gasped for air. His heart rate sped up. Eventually, the man had a heart attack and died.

The people who were watching asked the scientist, "What happened?"

The answer was simple. The human mind accepts whatever it believes, whether it's good or bad. It all depends on what you believe to be true.

Think about how many times we hear bad news, like being told we have cancer and that we're going to die. Will you believe it? Or will you stay positive and say, "I can beat this!"? It all depends on your beliefs.

Your mind is so powerful that it can either heal you or harm you. The choice is yours. Life is shaped by how you choose to see it, and positive thoughts can keep you strong. Even when life looks tough, remember that there's always a light shining through. Whatever doesn't kill you, makes you stronger.

We all see life in different ways, and we might not always agree. But what really matters is being there for each other when we need it the most. Our minds believe what we see, and we see what we believe.

The Power of Belief

My ancestors taught that the mind is a powerful tool, capable of shaping reality and influencing the body. Heritage wisdom from the custodians of the first nations emphasizes the deep connection between thought, spirit, and health, reminding us that our beliefs are as vital as the air we breathe.

The Mind as a Creator

The old ways teach that what we focus on becomes our reality. Just as the Earth shapes landscapes with its elements, the mind shapes our experience through thoughts and perceptions. Whether a thought brings healing or harm depends on the energy we give it.

The Interplay of Body and Spirit

The teachings of the ancestors highlight the unity of the physical and the spiritual. A belief held strongly enough can influence the body's health and vitality, as if the spirit speaks directly to the cells. This sacred connection calls us to be mindful of the stories we tell ourselves.

The Choice of Perspective

Life offers challenges, but the way we perceive them determines their impact. Choosing to see difficulty as an opportunity for growth reflects the wisdom of the old ways, which teach resilience and faith in the face of adversity. By focusing on light even in darkness, we align ourselves with the energy of renewal.

Community and Support

Sacred traditions remind us that no one walks the path alone. Surrounding ourselves with those who uplift and encourage strengthens our beliefs in healing, hope, and possibility. Just as a tribe thrives through unity, so does the individual through connection and shared strength.

Harnessing the Mind's Power

The teachings emphasize practices that align the mind with positive energy:

Gratitude: Giving thanks for life's blessings focuses the mind on abundance.
Affirmations: Repeating positive truths reinforces belief in healing and strength.
Visualization: Envisioning health and well-being helps guide the body toward balance.

Belief as a Sacred Gift

The ancestors viewed belief as a sacred power, one that could transform hardship into strength and fear into courage. By choosing beliefs that serve our highest good, we honor this gift and align ourselves with the greater harmony of life.

As the elders say, "The mind is the weaver of the spirit's tapestry." Let us weave thoughts of strength, healing, and light, remembering that our beliefs are the seeds from which our reality grows.

Mind-Altering Herbs

Have you ever gotten up from your chair, walked into another room, and stood there wondering, "What did I come in here for?" Then you turn around, walk back to where you started, and suddenly remember—"Oh, I forgot my glasses!" Back you go to get them.

If this sounds familiar, you're not alone. And guess what? It happens more often as we get older. Some people call these "senior moments," but I like to call them veinte vueltas—which means "20 turns"—because on a bad day, it can feel like you've been going in circles all day without accomplishing anything.

Or how about this? You carefully put something away for safekeeping, only to forget where you put it later. Frustrating, right?

Another common one is when you're mid-conversation with someone and suddenly forget what you were saying. You ask, "What was I talking about?" but they either don't remember or weren't paying attention because the conversation wasn't exactly gripping.

Most of the time, we blame these moments on being tired, having "brain fog," or needing caffeine. But be careful about what you use to wake up your brain. Not all over-the-counter pills are safe. It's important to read labels, research ingredients, and even question prescriptions your doctor might recommend.

Personally, I prefer natural remedies—herbs I can grow in my own garden. That way, I know they're fresh and free from any harmful additives. Thankfully, there are several herbs that can naturally support memory and brain health.

Top 5 Mind-Boosting Herbs

Drinking tea made from these herbs once or twice a day can help sharpen your memory and improve your focus over time:

Ashwagandha

This powerful herb protects your brain from cell degeneration. It's packed with natural antioxidants and plant-based steroids that improve brain function and overall health.

Rosemary

Known as the "herb of remembrance," rosemary improves concentration and memory. It stimulates circulation, bringing more oxygen to the brain for better focus and clarity.

Rhodiola Rosea

This herb is excellent for mental clarity and memory. It also helps reduce fatigue and anxiety, making it a great option for those high-stress days.

Lion's Mane Mushroom

Lion's Mane is a superstar for brain health. It enhances memory, slows down, and even reverses cell degeneration in the brain. This mushroom also stimulates the nervous system, which is essential for your body's overall health.

Turmeric

Turmeric is a powerful anti-inflammatory that improves brain function. It boosts levels of brain-derived neurotrophic factor (BDNF), a protein that supports memory and learning. When BDNF levels drop, forgetfulness and mental fog can increase.

Why Choose Natural Remedies?

Our bodies benefit from plants in countless ways, and using them helps us stay as healthy as possible. Yes, natural remedies may take some time to work, but they come without the risks of artificial additives or chemicals. Plus, you can adjust how much you use and even add a bit of honey to your tea for sweetness.

Taking these herbs is like giving your brain a little hug. Over time, you might find your memory improving, and you could even surprise yourself by remembering where you hid that special gift! Not only will you impress the people you love, but you'll also feel a sense of accomplishment—and that's a win-win.

So, take a moment to brew a warm cup of herbal tea, sit back, and let these plants work their magic. Who knows? The opportunities for a sharper mind and healthier brain are endless.

Nurturing the Mind Naturally

In the teachings of the ancestors, plants are seen not just as resources but as sacred allies—gifts from the Earth that nurture the body, mind, and spirit. Ancient teachings from the echoes of the original people emphasizes the deep connection between humans and nature, reminding us that the remedies we seek often lie in the plants that surround us.

The Mind as a Sacred Space

The old ways teach that the mind is a powerful and sacred space, deserving of care and attention. Moments of forgetfulness or mental fog are not failures but signals from the body, inviting us to slow down, reflect, and restore balance. Through the use of natural remedies, we can honor this call and support the mind's natural clarity and vitality.

The Healing Power of Plants

The ancestors understood that every plant holds unique gifts, offering healing properties that align with the rhythms of the Earth and the human body. Herbs that support mental clarity and memory are a testament to the harmony between nature and our own well-being. By incorporating these gifts into daily life, we reconnect with the wisdom of the natural world.

Patience and Trust in Nature

Unlike quick fixes, natural remedies work gently and holistically, aligning with the body's rhythms. This process requires patience and trust—qualities that the ancestors valued deeply. Just as a seed takes time to grow into a thriving plant, the benefits of natural herbs unfold over time, offering lasting support and balance.

Honoring the Cycle of Life

The old ways remind us that life is a cycle of remembering, forgetting, and relearning. Plants that enhance memory and clarity mirror this cycle, helping us to navigate the ebb and flow of mental sharpness. By embracing these remedies, we honor the interconnectedness of all things and our place within the greater circle of life.

A Ritual of Care

Preparing and consuming herbal remedies can be a ritual of care, a moment to pause and reconnect with oneself. Whether brewing a tea, inhaling the aroma of an herb, or reflecting on its origins, this practice deepens our relationship with the Earth and its gifts.

As the elders teach, "The Earth provides what we need, if only we take the time to listen and learn." By embracing the wisdom of plants and the gentle power of nature, we nurture not only the mind but also the spirit, fostering a life of clarity, balance, and gratitude.

Imagine Yourself Thin

Have you ever looked in the mirror and tried to picture a thinner, healthier version of yourself? Or maybe you've held onto a beautiful outfit, hoping that one day you'd be able to wear it again once you reached your goal weight. I used to do the same thing.

But over time, I realized something: holding onto those hopes without making real changes wasn't going to make that dream come true.

The Turning Point

I was the person who had always been overweight. As I got older, my weight became a constant struggle. But then, I discovered something powerful: changing the way you think about yourself and food can work wonders.

I began to look at food differently. Imagine you're at a restaurant, and you've just ordered dessert—a decadent chocolate pie with whipped cream. You've been thinking about this dessert all day, imagining how creamy and heavenly it will taste.

Now, when it's placed in front of you, what are your thoughts?

"Oh my gosh, this tastes like heaven!"
"Through my lips, forever on my hips."

If you chose the first thought, you're on the right track! Positive thinking sets the tone for how we approach food and life. But if you picked the second, that's okay—it just shows where a shift in mindset can help.

The Power of Positive Thinking

I started telling myself things like, "I can eat anything I want and still weigh 155 pounds." I stopped saying negative phrases like "This will make me fat" or "That has too many calories."

When I removed these negative thoughts from my mind, something incredible happened: I started losing weight.

Our minds are incredibly powerful. When we approach life with positivity and visualize the future we want, we can create that reality.

The Key: Moderation, Not Deprivation

I'm not saying you have to give up your favorite foods. In fact, you can eat them—all in moderation. But there's one critical thing to remember: never tell yourself you're on a diet.

Why? Because the word "diet" often triggers feelings of restriction. Suddenly, you start craving foods you didn't even think about before. Instead, focus on eating mindfully.

Here's a simple trick I used: tell your body, "Take the nutrients it needs from this food and get rid of the rest." Once you feel full, stop eating.

Letting Go of Guilt

Growing up, I heard the classic line: "Finish everything on your plate; there are starving children who don't have any food." But I learned to let go of the guilt of leaving food on my plate. It's not wasteful if your body doesn't need it—it's just being kind to yourself.

My Transformation

At my heaviest, I weighed 360 pounds. Using these simple methods, I lost the weight and kept it off. When my family saw the new me, they couldn't believe it. In fact, one of my uncles asked my sister if I was dying because he had never seen me so thin before!

Believe in Yourself

The key to lasting change is believing in yourself. Picture the future you want. See yourself healthy, happy, and vibrant. When you think positively, treat food with respect, and stay mindful, your body will follow suit.

Remember, this isn't about being perfect. It's about being kind to yourself, enjoying life, and making choices that bring you closer to the person you want to be. You've got this.

The Power of Vision

The wisdom of the old ways teaches that transformation begins within. Time-honored knowledge from the elders of the sacred traditions emphasize the strength of the mind, the importance of self-respect, and the deep connection between the body, mind, and spirit. Achieving balance and health is not about restriction but about honoring the sacred relationship we have with ourselves and the world around us.

Seeing Yourself Whole

Transformation starts with how you see yourself. Just as the ancestors would envision a harmonious future before taking action, we too must begin by picturing the version of ourselves that aligns with health, strength, and happiness. This vision becomes the guide that leads us toward balance, reminding us of the possibilities that await.

The Power of Positive Thought

The old ways teach that thoughts are seeds, and what we nurture in our minds will grow. By replacing negativity with affirmations of strength and capability, we align our energy with growth and change. Instead of focusing on what we lack or fear, we are called to celebrate what we are capable of achieving.

Food as a Sacred Gift

In indigenous traditions, food is seen as a sacred gift from the Earth. Eating mindfully and with gratitude transforms meals into ceremonies of nourishment and respect. It is not about deprivation but about balance, choosing foods that honor both the body's needs and the spirit's joy.

Listening to Your Body

The ancestors often spoke of listening—not only to others but to oneself. By tuning in to the body's signals of hunger, fullness, and energy, we cultivate a deeper understanding of what it needs to thrive. This practice fosters a compassionate relationship with the body, free of guilt or judgment.

Letting Go of Shame

Shame has no place in the journey toward balance. Heritage insights remind us that every step, even those that feel like setbacks, is part of the path. By releasing guilt and embracing self-compassion, we create space for growth and resilience.

Transformation as a Sacred Journey

Change is not a single act but a journey of small, intentional steps. Like planting a garden, it requires patience, care, and trust in the process. Each choice we make, whether to move our bodies, nourish ourselves, or think positively, is a step toward the thriving, vibrant life we envision.

As the elders say, "The path is made by walking." By embracing the power of vision, gratitude, and mindful choices, we honor the journey toward balance and celebrate the sacred relationship between the body, mind, and spirit. Let us walk this path with courage, joy, and self-love.

What You Can Do About Brain Fog

Have you ever walked into a room and then stopped, looking around and wondering, "Why did I come in here?" You might go back to the living room or kitchen and suddenly remember, "Oh yeah, I came to get my glasses!" Then you head back to the room, only to forget again what you needed. It can be pretty funny, but also a little frustrating!

Many people think this forgetfulness is a sign of getting old. But guess what? It can happen to anyone, even kids! Sometimes, it's because of things like not sleeping well, feeling very tired, or changes in our bodies. This feeling is often called brain fog.

What Is Brain Fog?

Brain fog isn't a real medical term, but it's a way to describe when our thinking feels fuzzy or cloudy. It's like when you're trying to watch a movie, but there's fog on the screen—you can't see clearly.

Signs of Brain Fog

How do you know if you're experiencing brain fog? Here are some signs:

- Low Energy: You feel tired even if you haven't done much.
- Feeling Tired: No matter how much you rest, you still feel sleepy.
- Frustration: You get annoyed easily because things aren't clear.
- Lack of Mental Clarity: It's hard to think straight or focus.
- Slow Understanding: Learning new things takes more time.
- Trouble Making Decisions: Even small choices seem hard.
- Forgetting Conversations: You can't remember what you just talked about.
- Getting Lost While Driving: You forget where you're going.

Why Do We Get Brain Fog?

There are many reasons why brain fog happens. Let's explore some of them:

1. Not Enough Sleep
If you're not sleeping well or staying up too late, your brain doesn't get the rest it needs.

2. Medications
Some medicines can make your thinking a bit cloudy. If you think this is happening, talk to a doctor.

3. Feeling Very Tired (Fatigue)
When your body is super tired, it can hardly work anymore. This makes it hard for your brain to focus.

4. Changes in Body Chemistry
Sometimes, changes inside our bodies can cause brain fog. For example:
- Hormonal Changes: Like during pregnancy.
- Chemotherapy: Treatment for cancer can affect your thinking.

5. Inflammation in the Body
Inflammation means parts of your body are swollen or irritated. Conditions that can cause this include:
- Lupus
- Allergies
- Arthritis
- Diabetes

6. Dehydration
Not drinking enough water can cause brain fog and even headaches like migraines.

7. Lack of Important Nutrients
Not getting enough vitamins and minerals, like Vitamin B-12 and magnesium, can make it hard for your brain to work properly.

How Can We Improve Our Thinking?

Now that we know some reasons for brain fog, let's see what we can do to feel better!

1. Talk to a Doctor
First, it's important to check with a doctor to make sure everything is okay. They can help find out if there's a medical reason for your brain fog.

2. Get Plenty of Sleep
- Aim for 8 Hours: Try to sleep at least eight hours each night.
- Relax Before Bed: Take a warm bath or shower to relax.
- Listen to Soft Music: Calming music can help you fall asleep.

3. Eat Healthy Meals
Your brain needs good food to work well!
- Omega-3 Fatty Acids: Found in fish like salmon, these help your brain.
- Healthy Fats: Avocados and walnuts are great choices.
- Lots of Veggies and Fruits: Leafy greens and colorful fruits have vitamins and antioxidants.
- Stay Hydrated: Drink plenty of water every day.

4. Exercise Regularly
Moving your body helps your brain!

- Keep Moving: If you've been sitting, get up and stretch.
- Make It Fun: Dance around the house, chase your pet, or play a game.
- Family Time: Get your family to join in the fun.

5. Take Breaks from Screens
Too much time on TVs, phones, or computers can tire out your brain.

- Set a Timer: After 30 minutes of screen time, take a 10-minute break.
- Do Something Active: Use break time to move around.

6. Manage Stress
Feeling stressed can make brain fog worse.
- Meditate: Sit quietly and breathe deeply for a few minutes.
- Talk About It: Share your feelings with someone you trust.
- Do Things You Enjoy: Hobbies and fun activities can reduce stress.

Let's Move Together!
One of the best ways to clear brain fog is to get moving.
- Dance Party: Turn on your favorite songs and dance like nobody's watching!
- Play Outside: Ride a bike, play tag, or toss a ball.
- Family Fun Time: Announce to your family, "In ten minutes, we're turning off the internet for thirty minutes to have some fun together!"

Brain fog can be frustrating, but with some simple steps, you can help your mind feel clear again. Sleep well, eat healthy foods, stay active, and take breaks when you need them. And always remember to ask for help if you need it—you're not alone.

Clearing the Mind

The ancestors teach that the mind, body, and spirit are deeply connected, and balance among them is essential for clarity and well-being. When the mind feels clouded or heavy, it is often a reflection of imbalance—whether from lack of rest, nourishment, or harmony with the natural world. Indigenous traditions from the keepers of the primordial flame remind us to approach such moments with patience, self-awareness, and intentional care.

The Importance of Balance

The old ways emphasize the need for balance in all things. Just as the Earth's cycles depend on harmony, so too does the mind rely on the balance of rest, nourishment, and activity. When this harmony is disrupted, the mind may feel foggy or unfocused, signaling the need to realign with the rhythms of life.

Listening to the Body's Signals

Brain fog is not a flaw but a message. It invites us to pause and reflect on what our bodies need. Perhaps it is rest after too much strain, water to quench thirst, or movement to awaken energy. By honoring these signals, we show respect for the wisdom of the body and its ability to guide us toward healing.

Nourishment for the Mind and Spirit

The teachings of the ancestors highlight the importance of feeding not just the body but also the mind and spirit. Fresh, wholesome foods, calming moments in nature, and joyful activities all contribute to mental clarity. When we nourish ourselves in these ways, we restore the energy needed for focus and creativity.

The Power of Movement and Stillness

Movement and stillness each play a role in clearing the mind. Gentle activity, such as walking or dancing, invigorates the body and brings fresh energy to the mind. Stillness, through practices like meditation or quiet reflection, calms the spirit and allows space for clarity to return. Together, they create the balance that fosters a clear and focused mind.

Connection with Nature

In traditional knowledge, nature is a source of healing and renewal. Spending time outdoors, feeling the wind, listening to water, or walking barefoot on the earth can help clear mental fog and restore harmony. Nature's rhythms remind us of our own need for flow and connection.

Caring for the Whole Self

The ancestors teach that care for the mind begins with care for the whole self. This includes:

- Sleep: Honoring the need for deep, restorative rest.
- Food and Water: Choosing nourishing foods and staying hydrated.
- Community: Sharing moments of joy and support with loved ones.
- Mindfulness: Being present in the moment and embracing gratitude.

Finding Clarity Together

Moments of fogginess are opportunities to slow down and reconnect—with ourselves, our loved ones, and the natural world. By embracing these moments with gentleness and wisdom, we create a path back to clarity and balance.

As the elders say, "The mind clears when the heart listens." Let us listen deeply, honor the needs of our body and spirit, and walk gently toward harmony and renewal.

Saying Thank You to Your Body

We often say "thank you" to people who help us. Whether it's carrying a bag of groceries, cooking a meal, or cleaning the house, we show our appreciation with kind words. Many of us also thank God for giving us another day of life, which is so important.

But have you ever taken a moment to say thank you to your own body for everything it does for you?

Why Thanking Your Body Matters

It might feel a little strange at first, but there's nothing wrong with thanking your body. In fact, it shows that you love and appreciate yourself. Just like talking to your plants helps them thrive, talking kindly to your body can make a big difference.

Your thoughts about yourself are powerful. Positive thoughts can bring happiness and self-acceptance, while negative ones can bring unnecessary pain.

Think about it: If you focus on what you don't like about yourself, you might believe that everyone else notices those things too. But the truth is, most people don't see what you see unless you point it out.

The Trap of Negative Thinking

We all have things we wish were different about ourselves. Maybe a woman feels insecure about her small breasts, or a man feels bad about his skinny arms. Maybe you've worried about losing your hair or something else about your appearance.

Sometimes, we try to "fix" what we don't like. While this can work out, there are also stories of regret—like when a surgery doesn't go as planned or someone looks back and realizes they were beautiful just as they were.

How often do people look at old photos and think, "What was I so worried about? I was gorgeous!" or "I was really handsome!"?

Remember, people who criticize your looks are often struggling with their own insecurities. Some might say hurtful things out of jealousy, while others may try to bring you down because they feel bad about themselves. These toxic people can affect your self-esteem, but you don't have to let their negativity define you.

You Are Beautiful in God's Eyes

You are a child of God, and He loves you unconditionally. In His eyes, you are beautiful just as you are. Lift yourself up and see the beauty within. Give thanks to your body for everything it does for you each and every day.

Your eyes let you see the world around you. Your lungs allow you to breathe, even if it's sometimes challenging. When you thank your body for these incredible functions, you might notice that you start to feel better.

Speaking positively to yourself isn't just about words—it's about transforming the way you see yourself.

Protect Yourself from Negativity

If someone says something negative to you, ask them to stop. If they don't, walk away. You don't need that kind of energy in your life. Surround yourself with people who lift you up, not tear you down.

Practice Self-Love

One powerful way to build self-love is to look in the mirror and say, "I love you." At first, it might feel awkward, but keep doing it. Every time you see a mirror, smile at yourself and say it like you mean it.

Tell yourself you're beautiful. Believe it. Speak kindly to yourself and watch how it changes the way you feel.

Gratitude for Your Amazing Body

Your body works hard for you every day. It fights off illnesses, heals from injuries, and keeps you going through thick and thin. Say thank you to your body for being there for you.

Practice gratitude and self-love daily. When you love and appreciate yourself, you'll see how truly amazing you are. You are strong. You are beautiful. And you are worthy of love—especially your own.

Honoring the Vessel: A Lesson in Gratitude and Self-Love

The teachings of the ancestors remind us that the body is a sacred vessel—a gift from the Creator, carrying us through life's journey. Indigenous traditions from the survivors of the ancient tribes emphasize the importance of honoring and respecting this vessel, recognizing it as an extension of the spirit and a connection to the Earth. Gratitude for the body is an essential part of living in harmony with oneself and the world.

The Power of Gratitude

Gratitude is a transformative force, capable of shifting perspectives and healing the heart. By expressing thanks to the body, we acknowledge the countless ways it serves us daily—the breath that sustains us, the eyes that witness beauty, the hands that create, and the heart that beats in rhythm with life itself. This simple act of appreciation strengthens our connection to our physical and spiritual selves.

The Harm of Negative Thoughts

The ancestors understood that words and thoughts carry energy. Negative self-talk can wound the spirit and create disharmony within. In contrast, speaking kindly to oneself nurtures strength and self-acceptance. Just as the Earth thrives under care and respect, so too does the body respond to loving attention and affirming words.

The Beauty of Imperfection

Ancient wisdom teaches that all things in nature, including the human form, are perfectly imperfect. Each wrinkle, scar, or feature is a story, a testament to the life we've lived. Instead of striving for an unattainable ideal, we are called to embrace and celebrate our uniqueness, knowing that our beauty lies in our authenticity.

Protecting the Sacred Self

The old ways emphasize the importance of surrounding oneself with positive energy. Just as a sacred space must be guarded against harm, so too must the self be protected from negativity. By distancing ourselves from hurtful words and people, and by welcoming those who uplift and encourage, we honor the sacredness of who we are.

Practices of Self-Love

The ancestors often used rituals to affirm life and connection. In the same way, simple daily practices like looking in the mirror and offering kind words can become powerful acts of self-love. Smiling at one's reflection, speaking affirmations, and expressing gratitude for the body are ways to strengthen the bond between the physical and the spiritual.

Synchronicity with the Body

When we honor the body as a sacred vessel, we align ourselves with the rhythms of life. Gratitude and self-love are not acts of vanity but acknowledgments of the divine within us. By caring for and appreciating our bodies, we cultivate harmony, resilience, and joy.

As the elders teach, "The body carries the spirit, and the spirit honors the body." Let us give thanks for this gift, treating it with the respect and love it deserves. Through gratitude and kindness, we become not only stronger but more connected to the beauty and wisdom of life.

Sound Therapy and Listening to Your Favorite Music

Karaoke, music, and sound can touch our hearts in amazing ways, often soothing our souls depending on the voice or melody. I didn't fully realize the power of singing until I gave it a try at my brother's house. He kept encouraging me to sing, but at first, I was too shy.

One day, I finally gave in—and I've never looked back. Now, I don't care how I sound, as long as I'm enjoying myself (though I still only sing with family, not in public!). I even sing to my granddaughter. She just smiles, and I like to joke that since she can't crawl yet, she has no choice but to listen.

Singing and music truly do the body good.

The Beauty of Music

There are so many kinds of music, each unique and beautiful depending on who is listening and what they enjoy. Some of the most popular types include:

- Country Music
- Rap
- Classical
- Mozart
- Drums and Rhythmic Beats

And that's just a start—there are countless styles and sounds to explore. No matter your favorite, there's usually that one song that takes you back in time the moment you hear it. Maybe it reminds you of a special dance, your first kiss, or just a favorite hangout where the music played in the background.

Music has a way of connecting us to memories and emotions.

The Science of Sound

Did you know that our bodies respond to sound in powerful ways? Our natural system of vibrations can be brought into balance through sound waves. This is the foundation of sound therapy, a practice that uses sounds and vibrations to help heal the body and mind.

For example, have you ever heard of singing bowls? These bowls, made of glass or metal, create soothing tones when played. Some people even place them on their bodies while they sing, feeling the vibrations flow through them.

Sound therapy has been shown to:

- Reduce stress
- Improve overall health
- Enhance emotional well-being
- Boost creativity
- Increase energy
- Improve brain function

It's also been helpful for:

- Young children with autism
- People with learning disabilities
- The elderly, especially those with Alzheimer's

How Music Matches Your Mood

Music can also change how we feel. If you're feeling down or stressed, try choosing songs that match the mood you want to feel instead of the mood you're in.

Feeling sad? Listen to upbeat music that makes you want to dance, like fun pop songs or rhythmic beats.

Need to relax? Try soft, slow tunes or even nature sounds like birds singing, creeks flowing, or ocean waves. (The sound of the ocean is my personal favorite, especially when I'm at the beach in person!)

The Healing Power of Music

Sound therapy isn't just about making you feel good—it can actually help your body heal itself. The vibrations in music connect to your body's natural rhythms, promoting balance and relaxation.

Sound therapy can:

- Help you relax
- Relieve stress
- Empower your body's self-healing abilities
- Support your overall health

Make Time for Sound Therapy

Whether it's through singing, listening to your favorite songs, or trying something new like singing bowls, sound therapy is a wonderful way to bring joy and balance into your life.

Let music soothe your soul. Dance, sing, or simply listen to the sounds that make you feel good. Remember, it's okay to let go, be happy, and live stress-free. Let the vibrations of music remind you of the beauty of life.

So go ahead—let the healing power of sound take over, and enjoy the rhythm of happiness.

The Harmony of Sound

In the wisdom of the ancestors, sound and rhythm are sacred tools that bridge the physical and spiritual worlds. Native traditions of the ancient custodians of the sacred wisdom teach that the vibrations of the Earth, the beat of a drum, and the songs of the people carry the power to heal, connect, and restore balance. Music and sound are not merely entertainment—they are living energies that touch the soul and align us with the natural rhythms of life.

The Spirit of Sound

The old ways remind us that sound is a gift, a form of energy that resonates deeply within us. Whether it's the steady rhythm of a drum, the soothing flow of a singing bowl, or the familiar melody of a favorite song, sound can awaken emotions, memories, and healing. Each note and vibration carries its own unique power, reminding us of the interconnectedness of all life.

Healing Through Vibrations

In traditional teachings, the body and spirit are viewed as harmonious systems of energy. When this harmony is disrupted, illness or imbalance may arise. Sound, with its ability to penetrate deeply, helps restore balance by realigning the vibrations of the body with those of the Earth. Practices like singing, chanting, and rhythmic drumming are powerful tools for healing, releasing stress, and nurturing the soul.

Music as Memory and Emotion

Songs carry stories, emotions, and connections to the past. The rhythms and melodies that resonate with us often hold the essence of shared experiences, bringing joy, comfort, or reflection. Ancestral wisdom teaches that these connections are sacred, reminding us that music is not just for the ears—it is for the heart and spirit.

Choosing Your Soundscape

The ancestors understood the importance of choosing sounds with intention. Whether to uplift the spirit, calm the mind, or heal the body, sound must align with the desired energy. Just as nature offers a symphony of soothing waves, rustling leaves, or birdsong, we too can select music or rhythms that nourish and balance us in the moment.

The Power of Singing and Expression

Singing, even imperfectly, is a form of self-expression and healing. The voice carries more than sound; it carries the energy of the heart. Whether shared in ceremony, with family, or alone in reflection, singing opens the soul and strengthens the connection between the self and the world.

Living in Harmony

The teachings of the old ways call us to live in harmony with the sounds around us. By embracing music and sound as tools for well-being, we honor their role in creating balance within and around us. Let the rhythms of life guide us toward peace, joy, and connection.

As the elders say, "The Earth sings, and so do we. Listen, and you will hear its song within your heart." Embrace the healing power of sound, and let its vibrations remind you of the beauty, balance, and unity that surround us all.

5 FOOD

Food has always been a big part of my life. It's not just about eating—it's about memories, connections, and even learning. I grew up believing that the food on our table was always good for us, especially the fruits and vegetables. But as I've gotten older, I've realized it's not always that simple. Some foods have hidden dangers, and others aren't as healthy as they seem. Still, I've found that knowing the risks doesn't mean giving them up; it means enjoying them in the right way.

Take tomatoes, for example. Who would think something so common could cause issues if you eat too many? Or kidney beans—they're a staple in so many recipes, but undercooking them can actually make you sick. Learning these things opened my eyes to how much there is to know about what we eat. It's not just about taste; it's about safety and balance.

In this chapter, I want to share what I've discovered about the foods we eat every day. Some of them might surprise you. Don't worry—this isn't about scaring you away from your favorite snacks or meals. It's about understanding how to enjoy them safely and wisely. Let's take a closer look at the foods we trust, the hidden risks they carry, and how a little knowledge can make a big difference in what we put on our plates.

Top 10 Most Dangerous Foods Your Mom Never Warned You About

Eating fruits and vegetables is supposed to be healthy, right? But some of your favorites might not be as safe as you think. It's not about avoiding them completely but knowing the risks so you can enjoy them safely. Here are 10 foods you should be cautious about:

1. Tomatoes

Tomatoes make so many dishes taste amazing, but eating too many can cause problems. They contain tomatine, a natural toxin, and may lead to inflammation or upset stomachs. They won't kill you, but moderation is key.

2. Cashews

Cashews are tasty, but did you know raw cashews are poisonous? They're covered in anacardic acid, which can be deadly. Luckily, roasting removes the poison, making them safe to eat. Fun fact: cashews are seeds, not nuts, and come from the cashew fruit!

3. Apricots and Cherries

These fruits are delicious, but their seeds are dangerous. They contain amygdalin, which turns into cyanide in your stomach if swallowed. That bitter taste in the seeds? It's nature's way of telling you not to eat them. Stick to the fruit and skip the pits!

4. Apples

"An apple a day keeps the doctor away"—but don't overdo it! Like apricots and cherries, apple seeds have amygdalin, which can turn into cyanide. Eating the fruit is fine, but avoid the seeds.

5. Asparagus

Asparagus is a healthy, delicious veggie, but beware of its bright red berries. They look pretty but are poisonous and can cause vomiting and diarrhea if eaten. Stick to the green stalks, and you'll be fine.

6. Kidney Beans

Kidney beans are common in chili, but eating them undercooked can make you sick. They contain phytohemagglutinin, which causes nausea, vomiting, and diarrhea. Make sure to cook them thoroughly before eating.

7. Rhubarb

Who doesn't love strawberry-rhubarb pie? Rhubarb's red stalks are safe and delicious, but its leaves contain oxalic acid, which can cause kidney failure and even death. Stick to the stalks—and the pie!

8. Pineapple

Pineapple is sweet and refreshing, but it's packed with sugar—about 16 grams per cup! Eating too much can harm your body. Enjoy it in small amounts to keep it healthy (and yes, it's great on pizza!).

9. Corn

Corn is a favorite in many forms—tortillas, popcorn, or corn on the cob—but much of it is genetically modified (GMO). Some worry these GMOs may not be good for us, so choose organic corn when you can.

10. Figs

Figs are sweet, delicious, and high in fiber, which can help lower blood pressure. But they also have about 16 grams of sugar per serving. While they're healthier than soda, eat them in moderation to avoid a sugar overload.

Stay Safe and Enjoy!

All these foods can be part of a healthy diet when eaten properly. Just remember to avoid the risky parts, eat in moderation, and enjoy their delicious flavors safely!

Well, here are some very good fruits and some vegetables that are very popular, yet not so safe to eat if we prepare them wrong or consume too much of. So, enjoy in moderation.

Bon Appetit!

Sugar Can Be Tricky

Almost everyone loves sugar, even if they don't realize it. It's everywhere—whether we choose it or not. Many foods either contain sugar or turn into sugar once we eat them.

Even if you're someone who avoids sugar, some of your favorite foods might surprise you. For example:

1. French Fries

French fries might seem savory, but they turn into sugar in your body.

2. Oatmeal

Oatmeal is a breakfast staple, but it also breaks down into sugar in your body.

3. Pizza

Who doesn't love pizza? Unfortunately, the dough and processed meats are unhealthy, loaded with calories, and contribute to sugar spikes.

4. Fruit Juice

Fruit juice is marketed as healthy, but it's often as sugary as soda. In some cases, it has more sugar than a can of Coke!

5. Cereal

Most cereals, even those labeled "healthy," are packed with sugar. Eating a bowl of cereal can be like eating candy with milk.

6. Pastries

Pastries may look delicious, but they're often made with unhealthy trans fats. Plus, they're full of sugar and often lack real flavor.

7. Gluten-Free Products

Many gluten-free products claim to be healthier, but the ingredients can still be packed with sugar or starches that turn into sugar.

8. Agave Nectar

Doctors often recommend agave nectar as a sugar substitute. However, it's even higher in fructose, which can harm your body.

9. Yogurt

Yogurt can seem healthy, but many varieties are loaded with sugar. If you stop eating sugar for a while, you'll be shocked at how sweet these "low-sugar" yogurts taste.

10. Diet Foods

Diet foods like low-calorie bars and frozen meals may seem like a good idea, but they're packed with additives and hidden sugars. Many people eat more of them because they think they're healthy, only to gain weight.

11. Processed Meats

Convenient for sandwiches or snacks, processed meats are harmful if eaten too often. They've been linked to colon cancer and heart disease.

12. Cheese

Cheese can be delicious in tacos or on burgers, but moderation is key. Beware of artificial cheeses with trans fats and fillers that mimic the taste of real cheese.

The Bigger Problem

Many of these foods are altered to make them cheaper or faster to produce. Companies use additives, fillers, and unhealthy ingredients without fully informing us. These changes can make us sick over time, but we rarely see clear warnings on the labels.

Take Action

Be mindful of what you eat. Read ingredient labels carefully, and try to choose fresh, whole foods whenever possible. Taking care of your health starts with knowing what's really in your food!

How Sweet Is Coffee Creamer?

Many of us love coffee with cream and sugar—it's hard to resist that creamy sweetness! I'm one of those people, though I've switched to heavy cream without sugar. Black coffee just doesn't do it for me.

I used to buy flavored creamers, but when I learned about the ingredients, I stopped. Both liquid and powdered creamers have some surprising (and unhealthy) additives. Here's what you should know:

What's in Coffee Creamer?
Powdered Creamer and MSG

Powdered creamers often contain MSG, hidden under the name "natural flavors." If they include soy, they can cause severe problems for people with allergies.

Dipotassium Phosphate

This ingredient is an anti-coagulant stabilizer found in non-dairy creamers. It's also used in cosmetics and fertilizer. Think about that the next time you stir it into your coffee!

Sodium Stearoyl Lactylate

This chemical is a cleansing agent used in cosmetics but also appears in powdered creamers to replace sugar and fat. Side effects may include:

- Stomach pain

- Nausea
- Headaches
- Vomiting

Trans Fats

Some creamers contain trans fats, which increase bad cholesterol (LDL) and can harm your heart. Trans fats are nearly identical to plastic on a molecular level, making them hard for your body to break down.

The Problem with Coffee Creamers

Liquid and powdered creamers are similar in terms of harmful additives. Over time, even moderate use can negatively affect your health, increasing bad fats and cholesterol. The FDA allows these ingredients, but they often go by confusing names to disguise their true nature.

For example, labels won't say "made with harmful chemicals" or "nearly plastic." Instead, they use scientific names most of us don't recognize. That's why it's important to read labels and look up ingredients if you don't understand them.

Healthier Alternatives

There's good news! You don't have to give up creamy coffee. Here are some healthier options:

- Plain milk with a bit of monk fruit sweetener
- Heavy cream for richness (my personal favorite!)
- Add a touch of honey for natural sweetness

If you're watching calories or trying to lose weight, you might want to go with plain coffee or limit creamers altogether. Everyone's tastes are different, so find what works for you!

Be a Smart Consumer

Many of us trust food companies without questioning what's in our food. However, these companies often hide harmful chemicals behind fancy names.

Before buying a product:

- Read the label carefully

- Use your phone to research ingredients

You may be shocked by what you find in your favorite creamer or other foods. Taking a few moments to check can protect your health and help you make better choices.

Enjoy your coffee but make it a choice that works for your body and well-being!

Are Eggs Good or Bad for You?

Are eggs healthy or harmful? This question has been debated for years, leaving many of us confused. First, experts said eggs caused high cholesterol, and then they changed their minds. So, what's the truth?

Here's what I've learned: Eggs are good for you! If they were as harmful as some say, we wouldn't see so many people thriving who eat eggs regularly. They're a staple food found in nearly every household. Let's break down why eggs are worth including in your diet.

The Benefits of Eggs

Packed with Nutrients

- Eggs are a quick and easy source of:

    o   Protein (6 grams per egg)
    o   Vitamins (like vitamin B and choline)
    o   Healthy fats (including omega-3s)

Boosts Good Cholesterol (HDL)

Eating eggs raises HDL cholesterol, which lowers your risk of heart problems.

Supports Brain Health

Eggs are rich in choline, an important nutrient for brain function. Just one hard-boiled egg a day can help your brain stay sharp.

Improves Eye Health

Eggs contain lutein and zeaxanthin, which reduce the risk of:

- Macular degeneration
- Cataracts

Good for Weight Management

Eggs help you feel full, making them an excellent choice for breakfast. They can keep hunger at bay until lunchtime.

Supports Muscles and Bones

The protein and amino acids in eggs help build muscle, strengthen bones, and maintain healthy blood pressure.

The Concerns About Eggs

There's a flip side, too. Some studies suggest eating too many eggs could lead to heart problems, as it may contribute to plaque buildup in arteries. While this concern existed for years, newer research shows that eggs are not the main cause of heart attacks.

The truth is, everyone's body reacts differently. For some, eating too many eggs might be harmful, while others can eat them regularly with no issues.

How to Eat Eggs Safely

To get the most benefits and reduce risks:

- Boil or poach your eggs instead of frying them.
- Eat eggs in moderation—one a day is a good starting point.

A Personal Perspective

I enjoy eggs in the morning and use them for baking. They're versatile, nutritious, and delicious. But like anything, moderation is key.

As my great uncle used to say:

"No matter how well we take care of ourselves, we all die someday. So, enjoy life and don't miss out on its simple pleasures."

In the end, the decision is yours. Listen to your body, consider your health needs, and enjoy eggs if they work for you. Life's too short to stress over every bite!

Using Herbs in Fruit Pies

Herbs are not just for teas or savory dishes—they can also make fruit pies extra delicious! I've always loved baking, but until recently, I never thought about adding herbs to pies. A friend of mine makes the most amazing pies, and after trying hers, I realized how much herbs can enhance the flavor of a homemade dessert.

Why Make Homemade Pies?

Store-bought pies, whether from the grocery store, bakery, or frozen section, just don't compare to a homemade pie. When you bake at home, you avoid preservatives, create something with love, and get so much more flavor. Plus, you can make healthier pies with fresh ingredients and a personal touch.

Adding Herbs to Pies

Adding herbs like sage, rosemary, or others can bring new layers of flavor to your pies. However, it's important to use herbs carefully so they don't overpower the fruit. Here are some tips to get started:

Start Small

- Use 1 teaspoon to 1 tablespoon of fresh or dried herbs, depending on their strength.

- Always taste as you go—it's easier to add more than to take it out!

Test the Combination

- Before adding the herb to all your fruit, mix a small amount with a little fruit and let it sit for 20 minutes.

- Taste it—if it's good, proceed. If it's not, you've saved the rest of your ingredients for another herb.

Chop Herbs Finely

For a smoother texture, chop fresh herbs very finely before adding them to the fruit or pie crust.

Add Herbs to the Crust

Mix finely chopped herbs into the flour before making your crust. This adds subtle flavor throughout the pie.

How Much Fruit and Herbs to Use

Use 5–6 cups of fruit for most pies.

Start with a small amount of herb and adjust as needed. Stronger herbs like rosemary might need less, while milder herbs like basil can handle a bit more.

Avoiding Mistakes

Using too much herb can make your pie taste like soap or stew—definitely not what you want! To avoid this:

- Always taste your herb and fruit mixture before baking.

- If the flavor seems off, try a different herb or adjust the amount.

A Lesson from My Baking Journey

When I first started experimenting with herbs in pies, I made small batches to avoid wasting ingredients. This way, if something didn't taste right, I was the only one who had to eat it. Nothing is worse than watching people grimace while trying to politely eat a pie that tastes like mouthwash!

Adding herbs to fruit pies can elevate your baking to a whole new level. Just take your time, experiment with small amounts, and enjoy the process. With fresh ingredients and a little creativity, you can create pies that are truly one of a kind.

Lessons from Food and Nature

The teachings of the ancestors remind us that food, like all aspects of life, is a source of both strength and caution. The natural world offers an abundance of nourishment, but it also carries lessons about balance, awareness, and respect. Sacred teachings from the unyielding spirits of the first lands speaks to the sacred relationship between humans and the gifts of the Earth, instructing us to approach food with gratitude, care, and mindfulness.

The Dual Nature of Nature

Everything in life holds a balance between benefit and risk. The ancestors understood that the same plant that heals can also harm if misused or misunderstood. This is a reminder to honor the natural world with respect and to take the time to learn about what we consume, whether it's herbs, fruits, or everyday staples.

The Importance of Moderation

In indigenous teachings, moderation is key to maintaining harmony. Foods that nourish in small amounts can overwhelm when consumed in excess. This principle extends not only to how much we eat but also to the energy and intentions we bring to the act of eating. Mindful consumption honors the balance between need and abundance.

Awareness as a Sacred Practice

The ancestors teach that knowledge is a form of respect. Knowing the properties of what we eat, how it is prepared, and the effects it may have is an act of care for both ourselves and the Earth. Whether avoiding harmful parts of plants or recognizing the hidden risks in modern foods, awareness strengthens our connection to the cycles of life.

Food as Medicine and Connection

Tribal wisdom sees food as more than sustenance—it is medicine, a bridge between the Earth and our bodies. Each fruit, herb, or vegetable carries its own spirit, offering unique benefits when approached with respect and understanding. This view invites us to see food not as a commodity but as a gift to be cherished.

Creativity and Gratitude

Cooking and preparing food can be an act of creation, a way to celebrate the abundance of the Earth. Adding herbs to pies, blending flavors, or finding healthier alternatives to modern ingredients reflects the joy and gratitude inherent in working with nature's offerings. These acts honor the Earth's gifts while fostering a deeper connection to our food.

Balance with Nature

The wisdom of the old ways calls for living in balance with the natural world. This means recognizing not only what the Earth provides but also our responsibility to protect and respect it. Choosing foods wisely, consuming mindfully, and appreciating their origins are ways to honor this sacred relationship.

As the elders teach, "The Earth gives what we need, but we must listen and learn." By approaching food with care, awareness, and gratitude, we not only nourish our bodies but also sustain the harmony between ourselves and the world around us.

6 BOTANICALS

Plants have always fascinated me. As a child, I loved exploring the garden, marveling at how flowers bloomed and leaves turned toward the sun. But as I've grown, I've come to realize plants are more than just beautiful— they seem to have a quiet wisdom, a way of sensing and responding to the world around them. Some people think it's silly to talk to plants, but I've seen how they thrive when they're cared for and appreciated. It's almost as if they can hear us—or maybe even feel the energy we send their way.

In this chapter, we'll dive into the mysteries of plants: their surprising abilities, their strength and adaptability, and their healing powers. From the way they seem to react to our emotions to the life-changing benefits they offer, plants have so much to teach us. Whether it's the basil in your kitchen, the cactus on your windowsill, or the trees in your neighborhood, every plant has a story to tell—and it's up to us to listen.

Can Plants Understand Us?

Have you ever wondered if your plants understand you when you talk to them? Well, they do—but you don't even have to speak! Just looking at them and thinking about how beautiful they are can make a connection. Plants seem to "read" your thoughts, just like pets such as cats and dogs can sense your emotions.

Do Plants Have Feelings?

It might sound unbelievable, but plants appear to have feelings and can communicate in their own way. Studies show that they react to their surroundings and even feel sorrow when other plants or living creatures are harmed.

Studies That Show How Plants React

Plants Feeling Sorrow for Fish

- In one experiment, scientists attached a lie detector machine to a plant's delicate leaf.
- In another room, a baby fish was dropped into hot water.
- The plant's reading on the machine was calm at first, but when the fish fell into the water, the needle spiked drastically.

This suggests the plant "felt" sadness for the fish's suffering.

Plants Reacting to Harm

- In another experiment, scientists connected a plant to a machine that could measure its energy.
- Nearby, a second plant was placed on the same table.
- A group of people passed by, and one person was asked to tear apart the second plant.
- The connected plant showed a terrified energy response when the second plant was harmed.
- Later, as the group walked by one by one, the plant's energy identified the person who had harmed the other plant.

The Strength of Plants

Plants might seem delicate, but they are incredibly strong and adaptable:

- They can break through cement.
- They survive in extreme climates, like scorching deserts or rocky mountainsides.
- They don't have the option to leave their environment, so they adapt to wherever they are.

What Can We Learn from Plants?

Plants are more aware than we might think. They can sense your thoughts and emotions, so be mindful of what you're feeling around them. Thinking happy, positive thoughts may even help them thrive.

Why Plants Matter

Plants do so much for us:

They supply the oxygen we need to breathe.

They are essential for the survival of all life on Earth.

We need to take better care of plants and their habitats. For example, places like the Amazon rainforest are irreplaceable, and destroying them harms the balance of nature.

A Reminder to Be Kind

The world depends on plants for survival. Let's do our part by protecting them, keeping them healthy, and showing gratitude for the incredible role they play in our lives. After all, plants might just be listening to us—and even reading our thoughts!

150 Varieties of Basil: Here Are the Top 6

Basil is a refreshing and fragrant herb. Its smell is as powerful as mint—just a little goes a long way! Did you know that centuries ago, people believed basil had mystical powers? It was often used in spiritual ceremonies because it was thought to have strong healing properties.

A Little Basil History

- Ancient Egyptians: Used basil in the embalming process.
- In Crete: Basil was planted around homes and temples to ward off evil spirits. It was also given to sweethearts as a gift.
- Later Misunderstood: Over time, people mistakenly thought basil was poisonous, so they stopped using it.

Basil originally came from Africa and Asia, thriving in hot, dry climates. That's why basil plants can struggle in colder conditions—something I learned the hard way when mine kept dying!

So Many Varieties

There are 150 species of basil, but not all of them are used in cooking. Some are hybrids used for landscaping or spiritual purposes. Basil plants cross-breed easily, which is why there are so many types.

The Top 6 Types of Basil

1. Sweet Basil

    o   This is the most common variety.

    o   Great for tomato sauces, soups, and pesto.

2. Lettuce Leaf Basil

    o   A type of sweet basil with larger leaves.

    o   Perfect for infusing oils or dipping bread. The flavor is so good, it might make your mouth water just thinking about it!

3. Genovese Basil

    o   Another sweet basil with a strong aroma.

    o   Commonly used in many dishes, especially Italian cuisine.

4. Dark Opal Basil

    o   Known for its beautiful deep purple color.

    o   Sweet-smelling and used in cooking sauces or even in flower arrangements to add fragrance.

5. Lemon Basil

    o   Tastes like lemon!

    o   Adds a citrusy flavor to salads, fish, and even sun tea.

6. Lime Basil

    o   Tastes like lime.

    o   Ideal for dishes needing a limey kick.

Easy Basil Syrup Recipe

This basil syrup is simple to make and tastes amazing. Here's how:

- Combine 1 cup sugar, ½ cup water, and ½ cup washed basil leaves in a small saucepan.
- Simmer until the sugar dissolves.
- Let it cool, then strain into a container.

This syrup keeps for about a week and can be used to sweeten tea, drizzle over fruit, or anything else you want to try. Be adventurous!

Growing Basil

Some of the basil varieties mentioned aren't sold in grocery stores but can be found at nurseries or gardening centers. Basil loves sunny spots and warm temperatures, so plant them where they'll get plenty of sunlight. Avoid the cold—it's not their favorite!

Now that you know more about basil, why not try growing or cooking with one of these varieties? With so many options, there's a basil for everyone!

The Top 12 Health Benefits of Cactus

I still remember when my mom used to cook cactus for my dad and uncle. She once gave me a taste, but I didn't like it at the time. Years later, I learned how amazing cactus is for health after meeting a woman who owned a bakery.

A Story About Healing

This woman told me she used to eat a lot of her baked goods because they smelled so good. Over time, though, the sugar made her very sick, and she was diagnosed with diabetes. She had to close her bakery for months to recover.

She visited an herbalist who told her to simmer cactus leaves and drink the slimy juice twice a day—once in the morning and once at night. She followed this routine for a year, and when she went back to the doctor, she no longer had diabetes! The doctors were amazed but didn't believe her when she explained how cactus had helped her.

This story shows how powerful cactus can be for your health. Known as the "humble plant," cactus has many benefits.

12 Amazing Health Benefits of Cactus

1. Helps Manage Diabetes

   o Drinking cactus juice regularly can lower blood sugar levels and help manage or even reverse diabetes.

2. Rich in Vitamins and Nutrients

   o Cactus is packed with essential vitamins, minerals, and nutrients that make it one of the healthiest plants to eat.

3. A Great Source of Fiber

   o Cactus adds a variety of fiber to your diet, which helps with digestion and overall health.

4. Lowers Cholesterol and Triglycerides

   o Eating cactus can reduce cholesterol and triglycerides, helping protect your heart.

5. Reduces Blood Sugar Levels

   o Regular consumption of cactus can lower blood sugar naturally.

6. Fights Cancer and Heart Disease

   o Cactus contains antioxidants like phenolics and flavonoids that protect healthy cells and slow the growth of cancer cells in the colon, liver, breast, and prostate without harming normal cells.

7. Protects Brain Cells

   o The fruit of the cactus has a compound called quercetin 3-methyl flavonoid, which acts as a powerful protector for brain cells.

8. Improves Digestion

   o Cactus enhances digestion, speeds up bowel movements, and reduces carcinogens in the digestive system.

9. Aids in Weight Loss

   o Cactus is low in calories, provides energy, and is rich in amino acids, vitamins, and minerals that help with weight management.

10. Reduces Inflammation

   o Cactus has anti-inflammatory properties that ease muscle pain, protect arteries, and help the cardiovascular and gastrointestinal systems.

11. Supports Skin Health

   o Cactus is full of electrolytes, antioxidants, and vitamins that protect your skin from sun damage and improve overall skin health.

12. Anti-Aging Benefits

   o Cactus fights signs of aging by enhancing collagen production, firming the skin, and improving elasticity.

Bonus Benefit: Dissolves Kidney and Gall Stones

Cactus fruit can also help dissolve kidney and gall stones. Simply blend the fruit with water and drink it regularly.

Cactus, also known as nopale, isn't just a plant; it's a powerful natural healer. Whether you're looking to improve digestion, protect your brain, care for your skin, or manage a health condition, adding cactus to your diet could make a big difference.

Next time you see cactus at the market, give it a try—it's nature's gift to health and wellness!

Mimosa Pudica – The Sensitive Plant

Have you ever heard of Mimosa Pudica, also known as the "sensitive plant"? When touched, its leaves instantly close up. It's fascinating to watch, almost like magic!

My First Mimosa Pudica

When I was about 7 or 8 years old, a kind neighbor gave me a Mimosa Pudica plant. He had a beautiful garden filled with flowers and vegetables and told me I could have the plant if I promised to take good care of it.

I was so excited to bring it home! My mom reminded me not to touch it too much because it could die. But being the youngest in a big family, no one listened. Soon, the plant died, and I felt terrible for not keeping my promise.

Finding the Plant Again

Years later, while working in a grocery store's flower department, I was watering plants when a drop of water fell on a small plant—and its leaves instantly closed! I was so thrilled to find the Mimosa Pudica again.

I brought it home and took great care of it. It grew beautifully, but then my sister-in-law got sick, and I had to leave town to help her. I asked my husband to care for the plant, but when I returned, it was dead. I was so disappointed.

My Search for Mimosa Pudica

Finding this plant again has been a challenge. For years, I described it to nurseries, but no one knew what I was talking about. I didn't even know its name until recently. Now that I do, I feel so much closer to finding it!

I once bought some seeds, but they didn't bloom because I didn't prepare them correctly. Now I know:

- Soak the seeds in warm water overnight.
- If they float, they're bad. If they sink, they're good to plant.

I just need to find the seeds again and try growing it properly this time.

The Healing Powers of Mimosa Pudica

Besides being a fascinating plant, Mimosa Pudica has amazing health benefits:

- Controls Blood Sugar and Blood Pressure
  - Helps regulate these levels naturally.
- Gut Health
  - Protects the intestinal tract and eliminates toxins.

- The seeds are known to protect against parasites.
- Pain Relief
  - Eases arthritis pain.
- Wound Healing
  - Speeds up recovery for cuts and injuries.
- Detoxification
- Cleanses the body of harmful toxins.

Why Mimosa Pudica Is Special

I always knew this plant was unique, but now I see just how extraordinary it truly is. Mimosa Pudica is not just shy—it's a powerhouse of healing potential for the body.

I'll let you know when I find the seeds and how my next attempt at growing it turns out. When I do, it'll be another thing checked off my bucket list.

The Spirit of Connection

The teachings of the ancestors remind us that all living things, from the smallest plants to the mightiest trees, hold a wisdom and energy that is deeply intertwined with our own. Sacred traditions from the eternal spirits of the Earth emphasize the sacred relationship between humans and the natural world, teaching that plants are not merely resources but conscious beings with whom we share a bond.

The Awareness of Life

The old ways teach that all life carries a spirit and a form of communication. Plants, in their stillness, are listeners, responders, and participants in the web of existence. Their reactions to their environment, their resilience, and their ability to heal and nourish reflect their awareness of the world around them.

The Power of Care and Respect

Plants thrive when tended with care, and their growth mirrors the energy and attention they receive. Whether through kind words, gentle handling, or mindful harvesting, the connection we build with plants is a two-way exchange. Respecting their life force, as the old ways instruct, allows us to access their full potential for healing and nourishment.

Lessons in Adaptability and Strength

From the cactus in the desert to the sensitive plant that responds to touch, the natural world teaches us about resilience and adaptability. Each plant holds a lesson about surviving and thriving in its environment. These teachings remind us of our own ability to adapt and grow, even in the harshest circumstances.

Healing Through Connection

Plants offer more than sustenance; they provide healing for the body, mind, and spirit. The ancestors understood that plants are gifts, each with unique properties to aid in human well-being. This sacred knowledge, passed down through generations, teaches us to seek out and honor the remedies the Earth provides.

Cultivating Gratitude

The wisdom of the old ways calls us to live with gratitude for the gifts of nature. Whether growing an herb garden, harvesting wild plants, or simply sitting in the presence of a tree, we are reminded to give thanks. This reciprocity strengthens our relationship with the Earth and ensures the continued abundance of its offerings.

A Shared Purpose

The stories of the ancestors often speak of humans and plants working together in harmony, each fulfilling a role in the circle of life. Plants, with their quiet strength and healing presence, are allies in our journey, reminding us of the interconnectedness of all beings.

As the elders teach, "The plants know the songs of the Earth. Listen, and they will teach you." By approaching the natural world with curiosity, respect, and an open heart, we nurture not only the life around us but also the life within us. Let us honor this sacred connection, learning from the plants as they guide us toward balance, healing, and harmony.

7 HERBALS

When I think about herbs, I'm reminded of the quiet magic they bring to our lives. Herbs aren't just for flavoring food—they're little powerhouses of healing, nourishment, and connection to the natural world. Growing up, I didn't fully appreciate the herbs my mom used in her cooking or the plants she carefully tended in our garden. But as I've learned more about their uses and benefits, I've come to see them as gifts from the Earth, offering so much more than just taste.

In this chapter, we'll explore some of the most amazing herbs and their incredible health benefits. From spices in your kitchen to the weeds in your backyard, these plants have stories to tell and healing to offer. Whether you're growing your own herb garden, using them in your meals, or discovering their ancient remedies, herbs remind us that the simplest things can make the biggest difference. Let's dive into their world and see what they can do.

Top 10 Herbs & Spices with Amazing Health Benefits

Adding herbs and spices to your diet doesn't just make food taste great—it also offers incredible health benefits. Here are 10 powerful herbs and spices you should know about:

1. Cinnamon

- Packed with antioxidants and anti-inflammatory properties.
- May reduce the risk of heart disease.
- Helps lower blood sugar levels, especially for diabetics.

2. Sage

- High in nutrients and minerals.
- Promotes brain health and improves memory.

- Helps regulate blood sugar and boosts heart health.
- Supports healthy skin and speeds up wound healing.

3. Peppermint

- Improves digestion and helps with colds and flu.
- Reduces fever and stress.
- Boosts mental awareness and prevents nausea.

4. Turmeric

- Contains curcumin, a powerful natural anti-inflammatory.
- Acts as a strong antioxidant.
- May help with skin problems and improve brain health.

5. Holy Basil

- Reduces stress, anxiety, and fatigue.
- Helps with arthritis and fibromyalgia.
- Taking holy basil oil can improve memory, sleep, and energy levels.

6. Cayenne Pepper

- Boosts metabolism and reduces hunger.
- Lowers blood pressure and aids digestion.
- Provides pain relief.

7. Ginger

- Brightens your smile and calms nausea.
- Eases arthritis pain and lowers blood sugar.
- Soothes period pain, lowers cholesterol, and relieves indigestion.

8. Rosemary

- Helps lower blood sugar and improves brain and eye health.
- Contains antimicrobial and anti-inflammatory compounds.

9. Garlic

- Loaded with nutrients that combat sickness like the common cold.
- Reduces blood pressure and improves cholesterol levels.

- Lowers the risk of heart disease and may even help you live longer.

10. Fenugreek

- Supports weight loss and helps nursing mothers with milk production.
- Boosts testosterone and sperm count.
- Lowers blood pressure and supports heart health.
- Naturally stimulates tissue growth, which may help enhance breast size without surgery.

A Word of Caution

Before taking any of these herbs as supplements, talk to your doctor to make sure they don't interfere with any medications you're on. However, when used in cooking, these herbs and spices add flavor and health benefits to your meals.

Without them, food—and life—would be much less exciting and healthy!

Most Used Herbs in the World

Growing up, I remember my mom's cooking always tasted amazing. With 11 kids to feed, though, getting seconds was rare. We were lucky just to get a full plate the first time!

Back then, I didn't think much about the herbs she used to flavor her dishes. As I got older, I relied mostly on salt and pepper in my cooking.

You might wonder, if my mom was such a great cook, why didn't I learn from her? Sadly, she passed away in a car accident when I was young, and with her went her cooking knowledge and herbal wisdom. My older sisters learned some of her secrets, but I didn't get the chance.

Rediscovering the Power of Herbs

Over time, I began learning about herbs from my sisters and others I met in life. I finally realized how much they enhance food and even help the body heal.

I do remember my mom grinding dried herbs in a molcajete (mortar and pestle). Back then, I didn't know what she was doing—she just told me to leave the kitchen so I wouldn't get in the way. Only my older sisters stayed to help.

Now that I'm older, I've learned to recognize herbs by their smells and associate them with their flavors. Here are four of the most popular herbs used around the world:

1. Cumin

Flavor: Warm and earthy.

Benefits: Aids digestion and is a rich source of iron.

2. Cilantro

Flavor: Strong and fragrant, especially when added fresh to food.

Benefits: Helps with digestion, fights infections, and improves sleep quality.

3. Garlic

Flavor: Pungent, sharp, and spicy.

Benefits:

Combats colds and sickness.
Lowers blood pressure.
Improves cholesterol levels.

Fun fact: Garlic can be eaten raw or cooked, adding bold flavor to any dish.

4. Oregano

Flavor: Strongly aromatic, slightly bitter, with earthy and minty notes.

Benefits:

Fights infections.
Helps with respiratory issues like cough, asthma, and bronchitis.

A Personal Story About Oregano

When my boys were little, they had bad mucus congestion in their lungs. You could hear it with every breath they took. I told a friend about it, and she shared an old remedy:

Make a tea using oregano and garlic.
Simmer it, let it cool, then add a little honey.
Give it to the kids and avoid dairy products.

I followed her advice for two weeks, and my boys' lungs cleared up completely.

Why Use Herbs in Cooking?
Using herbs in everyday cooking doesn't just add flavor—it also helps your body heal and fights off illness.

With so much processed food available today, cooking fresh at home with herbs is one of the healthiest things you can do for yourself and your family.

Herbs like these not only make your food taste better but also bring natural healing into your meals. Give them a try—you won't regret it!

Herbs for Energy and Alertness

Life today can feel like a constant rush. While some of us are always on the go, others find themselves stuck in a more sedentary routine, especially with modern technology taking over our lives.

How Life Has Changed

There was a time when we spent our days outdoors, enjoying the sun, playing, running, and living life to the fullest. Now, times have changed. Many kids don't play outside anymore. Instead, they stay glued to laptops, cell phones, or TVs.

This behavior isn't just limited to kids. As adults, we've become overly dependent on technology too. We've traded face-to-face conversations for texting and social media, creating a gap in our relationships with family and friends.

Why Energy and Focus Matter

This tech-heavy lifestyle also takes a toll on our bodies. Many of us deprive ourselves of sleep, pushing to stay awake and productive, but this only harms our health. To stay alert and energized, it's essential to get plenty of rest. Once you're well-rested, certain herbs can help improve focus, energy, and mood.

Here are some of the best herbs for staying awake and alert:

1. Rhodiola Rosea

Helps regulate your mood.
Improves concentration and reduces stress in the body.

2. Rosemary

Acts as a brain tonic, boosting concentration.
Increases oxygen flow to the brain, keeping you alert.

3. Ginseng

Known for boosting energy.
Stimulates the brain and helps maintain focus.

4. Sage

Enhances memory and lifts your mood.
Provides a gentle boost for mental clarity.

5. Peppermint

Inhaling peppermint oil or its aroma can:
Boost energy levels.
Improve alertness and mood.

6. Ashwagandha

Used for thousands of years.
Supports brain health, improves memory, and promotes better sleep.

7. Centella Asiatica (Gotu Kola)

Improves brain function and alertness.
Enhances mood and mental clarity.

Choosing the Right Herb

Each of these herbs offers unique benefits. If you try one and experience an allergic reaction, don't worry—there are plenty of other options to explore.

Always listen to your body and find the herb that works best for you.

By combining plenty of rest with the right herbal support, you can stay energized, focused, and ready to tackle your day!

The Herb Fenugreek

Many people today are unhappy with their bodies. Some turn to expensive and painful surgeries, like breast enlargements or butt enhancements, hoping it will make them feel better. But what if there were a natural, affordable, and painless solution?

The truth is, nature provides many powerful herbs that can heal and improve the body naturally. Unlike synthetic drugs, herbs work harmoniously with our bodies without the long list of side effects that often come with medications.

One such amazing herb is Fenugreek. Let's explore what it can do!

What Is Fenugreek?

Fenugreek is an herb with incredible benefits for both men and women.

Here are some of its uses:

For Men: Fenugreek helps boost testosterone levels.
For Women: It can increase milk production for breastfeeding mothers.
For General Health: Fenugreek reduces cholesterol, helps control appetite, and lowers inflammation.

Fenugreek for Natural Enhancement

Fenugreek is known for its ability to naturally enhance breast size. It works by mimicking the effects of estrogen and stimulating the production of prolactin, a hormone that promotes breast growth.

However, it's important to remember:

Once you stop taking Fenugreek, your breasts will return to their original size.

Always consult with a doctor or an experienced herbalist before starting any new supplement.

Taking too much Fenugreek can cause side effects like gas, bloating, diarrhea, stomach upset, or headaches.

Does It Work for Bigger Butts?

Fenugreek can also help enhance your buttocks, but you'll need to combine it with exercise to see noticeable results.

Fenugreek for Skin Care

Fenugreek isn't just good for your body—it's great for your skin too!

Deep Cleanser and Exfoliator

Crush Fenugreek seeds into a powder and use it as an exfoliant to clean pores and remove oil and dirt.

Anti-Aging Face Mask

Soak Fenugreek seeds in water overnight. Save the water—it works as a skin-tightening toner.
Grind the seeds into a paste and mix:
    1 tablespoon Fenugreek seed paste
    2–3 drops of lemon juice
    5 drops of rosewater
Apply the mixture to your face and leave it on for 5–10 minutes (longer if it doesn't irritate your skin).
Rinse off with warm water, and enjoy fresher, younger-looking skin!

Fenugreek is a powerful herb with many benefits, but it's essential to use it responsibly. Always do your research and consult an expert to make sure it's right for you. While it can't replace hard work and a healthy lifestyle, it's a natural way to support your health and beauty.

Are Weeds Healing Herbs?

Did you know that some of the "weeds" in your backyard are actually healing herbs? These plants, often overlooked or sprayed with chemicals, have amazing health benefits and can help your body in many ways.

Nature's Gift to Us

When God created the earth, He gave us plants to help heal and nourish our bodies. For centuries, people used plants to treat headaches, bleeding, broken bones, pain, and more. Sadly, much of this wisdom has been lost over time.

While some plant knowledge has been passed down, we now rely on modern technology to rediscover these natural remedies. By learning what vitamins and minerals these plants contain, we can figure out how they can help with various health issues.

Common Healing Herbs

Here are some everyday plants that can do great things for your health:

Chamomile

Helps you relax and sleep better.
Soothes colic and indigestion.
Brew it into a tea and add a little honey for sweetness.

Cinnamon

Tastes naturally sweet and makes a delicious tea.
Cassia cinnamon is especially helpful for controlling blood sugar.

Dandelion

Often seen as a weed, dandelion is packed with health benefits.
Helps with digestion and can even be used to make wine.

Be careful where you pick dandelions—avoid areas treated with chemicals.

Using Backyard Herbs

Many of these herbs are easy to find in your yard or at the grocery store.

Fresh herbs are the best, but if you can't find them, herbal stores are a great alternative.

Want to know if a plant in your yard is useful? Try this:

Take a picture of the plant.
Go online and visit sites like southernexposure.com to identify it.
Research the plant to learn its health benefits.
You might be surprised to discover that a so-called "useless weed" is actually a treasure trove of healing power!

The Next Step

Once you identify a plant, find out how it can help you feel better. Whether it's aiding digestion, improving sleep, or boosting your overall health, these natural herbs are a gift from nature.

So, the next time you see a weed in your yard, take a closer look—you might just have a goldmine of natural medicine growing right under your nose!

Knowing What Herbs to Grow

When planning your herb garden, it's important to think about what you want to grow and where. Some herbs come back every year (perennials), while others need to be replanted each year (annuals). Here's how to decide what's best for you.

Plan Based on Your Cooking

The type of herbs you grow should match the foods you cook most often. For example:

Mexican dishes: Grow cilantro, oregano, jalapeños, onions, garlic, and cumin.
Other cuisines: Choose herbs that fit your favorite recipes.

This way, you'll always have fresh herbs on hand for your meals.

Sunlight and Growing Needs

Some herbs need lots of sunlight, while others can tolerate shade. Check the sunlight needs for each herb and decide if they'll grow better in the garden or in pots that you can move indoors during cold weather.

Starting from Seeds or Plants

You have two options when starting your herb garden:

Buy Small Plants

Already grown in pots.
Easy to replant in your garden or larger pots at home.

Start from Seeds

More work but often more affordable.
Follow the seed packet instructions carefully.

Tip: Some seeds can be tricky to grow. If you've tried before and failed, don't give up! Look up detailed instructions online for extra guidance.

Preparing the Soil

Before planting, make sure your soil is ready:

Loosen the Soil

This helps water drain properly and allows roots to grow deeper.

Add Compost

Mixing compost into the soil provides nutrients and helps plants thrive.

Watering Your Herbs

Proper watering is key to healthy herbs:

Check the Soil First: Stick your finger a few inches into the soil. If it's still moist, wait a day or two before watering.

Avoid Overwatering:

Too much water can make plants feel "drowned," turning their leaves yellow and making them prone to disease.

Group Herbs by Water Needs: Plant herbs with similar water requirements together to make watering easier.

Growing herbs is a rewarding experience that can save money and make your meals more delicious. Whether you start with seeds or small plants, the key is to plan, prepare your soil, and care for your herbs properly. Don't be discouraged by setbacks—learning from mistakes is part of gardening!

Learning About Herbs

All herbs come from living things like plants, trees, flowers, roots, mushrooms, lichens, and more.

If you have a garden full of herbs, you're lucky—you can pick what you need whenever you want. But sometimes, you might need an herb you don't grow, which means taking a walk in the woods to find it.

Tips for Finding and Harvesting Herbs

When gathering herbs, preparation is key. Follow these tips:

Bring a Plant Guide

Use a book that shows the plant's growing cycles.
This will help you identify the plant correctly.

Know When to Harvest

Flowers: Wait until they are fully bloomed.
Seeds: Harvest later in the season when the seeds are ready.
Leaves: Pick after the morning dew has dried but before the sun gets too hot. This preserves the plant's essential oils.

Handle with Care

Cut small branches or leaves gently to avoid damaging the plant.
If you need the root, leave some leaves so the plant can keep growing.

Respect the Plant

Only take what you need.
Leave enough for the plant to recover and continue growing.

Lessons from My Mother

I remember my mother planting and harvesting herbs. One day, I asked her what she was doing and if I could help. She explained how to plant and use the herbs:

Some were spices to add flavor to food.
Others were medicine, like for a tummy ache.

Although I learned a little back then, I wish I had taken the time to learn more. Now that she's gone, much of her knowledge is lost.

Don't Miss the Opportunity

If you have a loved one who knows about healing herbs, don't let that knowledge disappear. Start a conversation:

Ask about the names of the plants and how to identify them.
Learn what parts of the plant to use and how to prepare them.
Find out if the herb is for external or internal use and what symptoms it can help heal.
Take notes and listen closely—you'll be amazed at how much they are willing to share.

Herbal wisdom is a gift that connects us to nature and to those who came before us. Don't wait until it's too late to learn from the people who have this knowledge. You'll treasure what you learn forever.

Wisdom in Growing and Gathering

The teachings of the ancestors remind us that tending to the land is not just an act of cultivation but a form of relationship. In the traditions of indigenous cultures, each plant carries a spirit and purpose, offering gifts to those who approach with respect and care. An herb garden, whether cultivated at home or discovered in the wild, is a reflection of this sacred bond between humanity and the natural world.

Planting with Purpose

In the old ways, planting is done with intention. Herbs are chosen not only for their utility but for their alignment with the needs of the family and community. Just as we must care for the land, the land cares for us, providing flavors for nourishment and medicines for healing. Planning based on your needs, whether for sustenance or well-being, honors this reciprocal relationship.

Respect for the Earth

Every step of gardening and harvesting calls for respect. From preparing the soil to gathering leaves or roots, the Earth's gifts are not to be taken for granted. The wisdom of the old ways teaches us to take only what we need and to leave enough for the plant to thrive, ensuring its abundance for future seasons.

Learning from Elders and the Land

The knowledge of herbs is not just found in books but in the voices of those who have come before us. Indigenous traditions emphasize listening to elders, whose wisdom is a bridge to the past. By learning the names, uses, and preparation of plants, we honor their legacy and ensure that this knowledge continues to thrive.

The Harmony of Care

Tending to an herb garden or gathering in the wild is an act of harmony. Watering with care, grouping plants by their needs, and harvesting at the right time all reflect the rhythms of nature. These practices teach patience, mindfulness, and the value of nurturing life.

A Journey of Discovery

Herbalism is not only about results but about the journey of connection. The scents of the soil, the feel of leaves between fingers, and the joy of witnessing plants grow remind us of the beauty and simplicity of life. Each step deepens our connection to the Earth and to the wisdom it holds.

As the elders say, "The plants know what we need, but we must take the time to listen." By growing and gathering with intention, respect, and love, we cultivate not just a garden but a relationship with the Earth that nourishes the body, mind, and spirit.

8 WHATS THAT SMELL?

Have you ever walked by someone and caught a whiff of a fragrance so perfect that you couldn't help but smile? Maybe it made you wonder what they were wearing—or even wish you could smell that amazing too. Then, there are the moments when a scent is so strong or just doesn't seem right, and all you want to do is escape. I used to think finding the perfect scent was as simple as picking one I liked in the store, but I've learned that it's much more personal. The way a fragrance smells on you isn't just about the perfume—it's about your unique body chemistry and balance.

In this chapter, we'll explore why certain scents work beautifully on some people but not on others, and how understanding your body's pH balance and natural chemistry can help you choose a fragrance that truly complements you. Let's uncover the secrets behind "what's that smell?"— and how to make it yours.

Perfume, Smells, and pH Balance

Have you ever smelled someone and thought, Wow, they smell amazing! Maybe you even wanted to ask what perfume or cologne they were wearing. Then there's the person whose fragrance is so overpowering you can smell it before they even walk into the room, and you can't get away fast enough.

Why do perfumes and colognes smell great on some people but not on others? The answer lies in your body's pH balance. Your pH balance measures the acids and bases in your body, with 7.40 being ideal on a scale from 0 (acidic) to 14 (basic). The lungs and kidneys play a huge role in keeping your pH level stable, and when they're working well, your body is better able to harmonize with a fragrance.

Here's something interesting: oily skin makes perfume last longer, while dry skin causes it to fade faster. But even if your favorite fragrance smells fantastic on someone else, it may not have the same effect on you. That's because everyone's pH balance is unique—just like fingerprints. This uniqueness affects how scents react with your skin.

What Affects How a Fragrance Smells on You?

What You Eat: Foods like garlic, fish, and onions can alter your natural scent. When these odors mix with perfume or cologne, they can enhance or ruin the fragrance.

Health and Lifestyle: If you spray perfume and can't smell it on yourself, it might be a sign your pH is off. A hangover can also affect your fragrance because your body is trying to flush out toxins and sugars through your pores.

Skin Chemistry: Your body's natural oils and pH balance create a unique reaction with fragrances, making them smell different on you than on someone else.

Tips for Choosing the Right Perfume or Cologne

Always try a scent on your skin before buying it. Spray it on and wait about 20 minutes to let the top notes fade and the heart and base notes develop.

Don't be in a rush. Give the fragrance time to react with your body chemistry to ensure it smells as good as you expect.

Remember, a scent that smells great on a test strip or someone else might not suit your unique chemistry.

Perfume Notes: The Layers of a Fragrance

Perfumes and colognes have layers called "notes." These notes unfold in phases, and each plays a role in how the fragrance smells over time.

Top Notes (Head Notes)

These are the first scents you smell right after spraying. They're light, fresh, and sharp but fade quickly. Examples: Citrus, lavender.

Middle Notes (Heart Notes)

These emerge as the top notes fade and are considered the heart of the fragrance. They're softer, more mellow, and define the main character of the scent. Examples: Jasmine, cinnamon.

Base Notes

These are the deepest and longest-lasting scents. They anchor the fragrance, giving it richness and depth. Examples: Vanilla, musk.

The magic of a perfume comes from how these notes interact. It's like a song, with each note transitioning smoothly to the next.

Categories of Notes

Top Notes: Light and refreshing (e.g., citrus, lavender).

Heart Notes: Floral and spicy (e.g., jasmine, cinnamon).

Base Notes: Warm and rich (e.g., vanilla, musk).

There are also combinations of scents like fresh florals, spices, woody aromas, and musk. Top notes often include fresh florals, while woody and musky scents are found in the base notes.

How to Make Sure a Fragrance is Right for You

When you're shopping for perfume or cologne, spray it on your skin and take your time. Let the notes fully develop over 20 minutes to an hour. By then, you'll know if it's the right match for your unique chemistry. Don't just buy a scent because it smells good on someone else—it might not work for you.

Sometimes, when you're at the store for an hour or two, you've already got the perfect amount of time to test a fragrance. Use your nose as a "scent detector." If the perfume still smells fabulous after an hour, it's likely a good fit. If not, it's better to walk away than regret your choice.

The right fragrance can make people want to know where that amazing smell is coming from, while the wrong one might have them avoiding you. Take your time, and you'll end up smelling as wonderful as you want to feel.

The Harmony of Scent: Lessons from Nature and Balance

The wisdom of the ancestors teaches that harmony and balance are the foundation of all things, including the fragrances we wear and how they interact with us. Indigenous traditions from the sages of the ancestral forests emphasize the connection between the body, the Earth, and the spirit, reminding us that the uniqueness of each individual reflects the diversity of the natural world.

The Essence of Individuality

Just as no two leaves are the same, every person carries a distinct essence shaped by their body's chemistry, lifestyle, and connection to the environment. Scents, like the plants and oils they are often derived from, are alive and respond to the unique energy and balance of the wearer. This interplay between fragrance and the body is a reminder of how deeply interconnected we are with the world around us.

Balance as the Key

Indigenous teachings often speak of the importance of balance—within ourselves and with the world. The body's natural equilibrium, reflected in its chemistry and energy, determines how external elements interact with us. Fragrance is no exception. When the body is in harmony, it can better complement and carry the subtle notes of scent, much like a well-tuned drum resonates with clarity.

The Layers of Experience

In traditional storytelling, meaning is often revealed in layers, with each part adding depth to the whole. Similarly, the experience of a fragrance unfolds in layers, from its initial spark to its lasting impression. The top, middle, and base notes of a scent mirror this progression, teaching patience and the value of allowing time for true essence to emerge.

A Thoughtful Approach

Choosing a fragrance is not unlike choosing plants for medicine or ceremony. It requires care, attention, and respect for the individuality of the elements involved. Testing, observing, and taking time to ensure harmony between the scent and the self honors the wisdom of patience and mindfulness.

Connection Through Aroma

The scents we wear are more than just adornments; they are expressions of who we are and invitations to connect. A well-chosen fragrance reflects the wearer's essence and can evoke feelings of warmth, comfort, or intrigue in those around them. However, as the ancestors teach, true connection is about balance and subtlety—not overwhelming others, but inviting them closer.

Resonating with the Connection

The old ways remind us that everything we take into our lives, from food to fragrance, should align with our natural state and enhance, not disrupt, our harmony. By embracing this mindset, we cultivate a deeper connection to ourselves and the world, ensuring that every choice we make resonates with authenticity and balance.

As the elders say, "The spirit of a thing is its truest gift." Whether in the scents we wear or the lives we lead, honoring the balance between essence and expression brings beauty and harmony to all we touch.

9 OTHER MODALITIES

Have you ever felt stuck, like no matter what you do, something just isn't clicking? I know I have, and those moments can feel overwhelming. But they can also be the perfect time to explore new ways to grow, heal, and find balance. That's where "other modalities" come in. These are alternative approaches—like Reiki, reflexology, homeopathy, or even life coaching—that focus on the whole person, not just the symptoms. They aim to restore harmony in your mind, body, and spirit in ways that traditional methods might not touch.

I've seen firsthand how these practices can spark real transformation. Whether it's the soothing energy of Reiki helping to calm stress, reflexology bringing surprising relief through pressure points on your feet, or the personalized healing of homeopathy, these modalities offer tools to help you feel more balanced, energized, and alive. They can complement medical treatments, support emotional well-being, and even guide you toward your life's goals.

In this chapter, I'll share stories, insights, and practical tips about these healing and supportive practices. Whether you're curious about energy healing, looking for natural ways to manage pain, or wondering how a life coach might help you move forward, you'll find inspiration here. Let's explore these fascinating methods together—you might just discover the missing piece that helps you feel more like yourself again.

The Ancient Art of Acupuncture: Pathways to Hidden Healing

Acupuncture, an ancient Chinese healing art, is one of the most profound contributions to holistic medicine. With roots stretching back thousands of years, it offers a unique perspective on health by recognizing the flow of energy—or qi (pronounced "chee")—through the body's intricate network of meridians. This practice has not only stood the test of time but has also inspired and influenced countless other healing modalities around the world, revealing hidden pathways to health, including connections to chakras, auras, and the body's energetic field.

The Foundation of Acupuncture

Acupuncture is based on the idea that the human body is an interconnected system of energy channels known as meridians. These meridians are believed to carry life force energy throughout the body, influencing physical, emotional, and spiritual health. When the flow of qi becomes blocked or unbalanced, it can lead to discomfort, illness, or emotional unrest.

By inserting fine, sterile needles into specific points along these meridians, acupuncturists aim to restore the free flow of qi. This balances the body's energy, promotes healing, and enhances overall well-being. The brilliance of acupuncture lies in its holistic view of the human being—not just as a physical body, but as an integrated system of energy.

Influence on Other Healing Modalities

Acupuncture's understanding of energy pathways and their influence on health has served as a foundation for numerous other modalities. These pathways have inspired deeper exploration into the body's subtle energy systems, including the chakras and auras, which are central to other healing traditions.

Chakras and Energy Centers The concept of meridians in acupuncture aligns closely with the chakra system, a cornerstone of Indian Ayurvedic and yogic traditions. Chakras are energy centers along the spine that correspond to different aspects of physical and spiritual health. Many practitioners now integrate acupuncture with chakra balancing, using needles to stimulate specific points that correspond to these energy centers.

For example, acupuncture points along the Du meridian (governing vessel) can align with the crown chakra, enhancing spiritual connection, while points on the Ren meridian (conception vessel) resonate with the sacral chakra, promoting emotional and creative flow.

Auras and Subtle Energy Fields Acupuncture also paved the way for understanding the human aura, the subtle energy field surrounding the body. By addressing disruptions in qi within the body's meridians, acupuncture indirectly influences the aura. Modern energy healers often combine acupuncture with practices like Reiki or sound therapy, recognizing the interplay between meridians and the aura's layers.

Reflexology and Acupressure Reflexology, which focuses on stimulating points on the feet, hands, and ears to promote healing throughout the body, draws heavily from acupuncture's mapping of the meridians. Similarly, acupressure applies manual pressure to acupuncture points, offering a needle-free alternative that still works with the body's energy pathways.

Energy Psychology Techniques Modalities like Emotional Freedom Technique (EFT), or "tapping," owe much to acupuncture's understanding of meridian points. By tapping specific points while addressing emotional distress, practitioners release energetic blockages and promote emotional healing.

Revealing Hidden Pathways to Healing

Acupuncture's influence extends beyond physical health—it also encourages exploration of the mind-body-spirit connection. Through the lens of acupuncture, we come to see health not as the absence of disease but as a harmonious flow of energy that encompasses all aspects of existence.

Mapping the Invisible By revealing the existence of meridians, acupuncture opened the door to a broader understanding of how energy moves through the body and the subtle fields around it. This understanding has helped validate practices like chakra alignment and aura cleansing, which were once dismissed by the Western medical model.

Integrating Modern and Traditional Healing Acupuncture bridges the gap between ancient wisdom and modern science. Techniques like electroacupuncture, which uses electrical stimulation on needles, demonstrate how traditional knowledge can evolve to meet contemporary needs. At the same time, acupuncture has introduced modern medicine to the importance of energy balance in health.

Promoting Self-Healing Acupuncture reminds us that the body has an innate ability to heal itself when given the right conditions. This principle underpins many other modalities, from Ayurvedic medicine to Reiki, and emphasizes the empowerment of individuals to take charge of their healing journey.

A Universal Gift to Humanity

Acupuncture's profound wisdom has transcended its origins, inspiring a global appreciation for the interconnectedness of life and the subtle energies that sustain it. It serves as a bridge between cultures and healing traditions, showing us that while the languages of healing may differ, the goals are universal: balance, harmony, and well-being.

As acupuncture continues to influence and integrate with other modalities, it reminds us of the importance of looking beyond the physical and embracing the unseen forces that shape our lives. Whether through needles, touch, or energy work, the pathways it reveals guide us toward wholeness—not just as individuals, but as part of the universal consciousness.

What is Reiki and How Can It Help You?

I'm a Reiki practitioner, and I'd like to share how Reiki could make a difference in your life. Reiki is a gentle form of energy healing that focuses on balancing the energy in your body, mind, and spirit. The word "Reiki" comes from two Japanese words: rei, which means "universal," and ki, which means "life energy." You can think of it as tapping into the natural energy that flows all around us to help you feel your best.

During a Reiki session, I use my hands to channel energy to different areas of your body. Sometimes I place my hands lightly on you, and other times I hold them just above your body. There's no pressure, no pain—it's completely relaxing. Many people describe the experience as feeling a warm, gentle energy flowing through them. Others say they feel deeply calm, like they're wrapped in a soft blanket of peace.

Reiki is incredibly versatile and can help with many things, including:

- Stress relief: Reiki helps calm your mind and body, making it easier to handle life's challenges.
- Physical healing: It can reduce pain, improve circulation, and support your body's natural ability to heal.

- Emotional well-being: If you're feeling overwhelmed, anxious, or stuck, Reiki can help you feel more balanced and uplifted.
- Better sleep: Many people find that they sleep more deeply and wake up feeling refreshed after a Reiki session.
- Spiritual growth: For some, Reiki opens the door to a deeper sense of connection and purpose.

One of the beautiful things about Reiki is that you don't have to believe in it for it to work. Just like the sun warms you whether you understand how it works or not, Reiki energy flows where it's needed. It works alongside any medical treatments or therapies you're already using, making it a safe and natural way to support your health.

For me, Reiki has been a transformative journey. Not only has it helped me find balance and calm in my own life, but it's also given me a way to share those gifts with others. I love seeing people leave a session feeling lighter, more relaxed, and more in tune with themselves.

If you're curious about Reiki, I encourage you to give it a try. Whether you're dealing with physical pain, emotional struggles, or just looking for a way to unwind, Reiki can help you feel more at peace with yourself and the world around you. Let's work together to bring some healing and harmony into your life.

What is Homeopathy and How Can It Help You?

Homeopathy is a natural system of medicine that has been helping people feel better for over 200 years. It's based on the idea that "like cures like," meaning a substance that causes symptoms in a healthy person can, in very small amounts, help treat similar symptoms in someone who is unwell. Homeopathy uses highly diluted natural substances, like plants, minerals, and animal products, to stimulate the body's natural healing abilities.

One of the things I love about homeopathy is how gentle and personalized it is. Homeopaths don't just look at the symptoms of an illness—they consider the whole person, including physical, emotional, and even mental well-being. For example, if you're dealing with a headache, a homeopath would ask questions about your lifestyle, emotions, and stress levels to find the right remedy for you.

How Can Homeopathy Help You?

Homeopathy can support a wide range of health concerns, such as:

- Chronic conditions: Arthritis, asthma, and allergies.
- Acute illnesses: Colds, flu, ear infections, or injuries.
- Emotional well-being: Stress, anxiety, and depression.
- General health: Boosting your immune system or helping you recover from surgery or illness.

One of the great things about homeopathy is that it's safe for people of all ages, including babies, pregnant women, and the elderly. Because the remedies are so diluted, there's little risk of side effects, and they can often be used alongside other treatments.

Interested in Becoming a Homeopath?

If you find homeopathy fascinating and want to help others using this natural approach, you might enjoy becoming a homeopath. Here are some steps to learn more and get started:

Research: Start by reading books about homeopathy or taking an introductory course. Authors like Samuel Hahnemann (the founder of homeopathy) and modern practitioners provide excellent insights.

Find a School: Look for accredited schools or online programs that teach homeopathy. Many countries have professional organizations that can guide you to reputable institutions.

Shadow a Practitioner: Spend time with a practicing homeopath to see how they work and whether it feels like a good fit for you.

Get Certified: Depending on where you live, you may need to complete a certification or licensing program to practice homeopathy professionally.

Join a Community: Connect with professional organizations, attend workshops, and network with other homeopaths to continue learning and growing in the field.

Why Choose Homeopathy?

For me, homeopathy is more than just a way to treat symptoms—it's a way to bring balance and harmony back into people's lives. Whether you're looking for natural remedies to support your health or considering a career helping others, homeopathy offers a gentle, effective approach that works in harmony with the body's natural healing processes.

If this resonates with you, I encourage you to explore it further. Whether you're a patient or a future practitioner, homeopathy can open the door to a healthier, more holistic way of living.

Reflexology: Healing with a Touch

Have you ever heard of reflexology? It's a way to help your body heal by massaging certain spots on your feet and hands. These areas are connected to other parts of your body through nerve endings, and when you stimulate them, you can feel better in surprising ways.

The best thing about reflexology is that you can use it to target the areas where your body needs healing. By massaging these points with your fingers or thumbs, you can unblock energy pathways and start the healing process. If you're feeling pain or discomfort on the right side of your body, you work on your right foot. For the left side, you massage your left foot.

Why Reflexology Works

Our bodies have energy pathways and zones that are connected to overall health. Reflexology focuses on balancing these energies to promote healing. It's been used to relieve many issues, like:

- Headaches
- Constipation
- Insomnia
- Sinus problems
- Stress

It can even improve blood flow, balance glands, and help you feel more relaxed.

How to Get Started

You can visit a certified reflexologist or learn to do it yourself at home. Reflexology maps show which areas of your feet and hands connect to different organs and parts of your body. For example:

The upper foot connects to the eyes, liver, and kidneys.

The sole of the foot is divided into 30 areas, each linked to a specific part of the body.

Reflexology Methods

There are two main techniques for massaging your feet:

Thumb Method

Use your thumb to slowly press along the sides of your foot.
Feel for knots or small hard spots—these are blockages.
Massage them gently to release tension. It might hurt a little, but the relief afterward is worth it!

Finger Method

Use your index finger instead of your thumb.
Hold the foot with one hand while you massage with the other.
Choose the method that feels most comfortable for you.

Hand Reflexology

Your hands also have reflex points connected to other parts of your body. For example:

The elbow links to the knee.
The wrist connects to the ankle.

You can massage these areas daily to help keep your body balanced and healthy.

Daily Practice for Wellness

Making reflexology a part of your daily routine can help your body stay in balance. When your body is balanced, it works better, and you'll feel healthier and get sick less often.

Take some time each day to care for yourself with reflexology. With just one touch in the right places, you can start feeling better and keep your body on the path to wellness!

Ayurvedic Medicine: A Path to Balance and Healing

Ayurvedic medicine is an ancient healing system that has been practiced in India for over 2,500 years. It focuses on understanding the connection between the human body and the universe, seeing the body as a smaller version (microcosm) of the larger world around us. The goal of Ayurveda is to maintain balance within the body and with the world.

The Five Elements

Ayurveda is based on five natural elements:

- Earth
- Air
- Fire
- Water
- Space (Wind)

Each person has a unique combination of these elements, but some elements may be stronger in one person than another.

The Three Doshas

The three doshas, or life forces, represent combinations of these elements. Together, they are called the "tri dosha." Each dosha influences a person's physical, emotional, and mental traits.

Vata (Wind and Space)

Represents movement, lightness, and energy.
Controls the flow of fluids and cells in the body, connecting them to the brain.

People with strong Vata are creative, artistic, and full of ideas. They love staying busy and quickly get restless if they're not active.

Pitta (Fire and Water)

Represents transformation and metabolism.
Responsible for digestion and turning food into energy.

People with strong Pitta are action-oriented, focused, and competitive. They don't wait around—they get things done!

Kapha (Earth and Water)

Represents physical strength and stability.

Provides structure, healing abilities, and calmness.

People with strong Kapha are steady, tranquil, and strong, both emotionally and physically, like a bear.

Your Dosha at Birth

The day you are born, your body receives its unique dosha makeup, called "prakriti." This balance keeps you healthy at birth, but as life goes on, stress, poor diet, and unhealthy habits can throw your doshas out of balance, leading to illness.

Staying Healthy with Ayurveda

Ayurveda focuses on prevention and balance. To stay healthy, practitioners recommend:

Eating moderately and avoiding overeating.
Getting plenty of rest.
Managing stress through techniques like meditation.

If your doshas become unbalanced, meditation and Ayurvedic remedies can help restore harmony. Remedies may include:

Spices to aid digestion and balance.
Minerals to strengthen the body.
Gems and colors for energy healing.
Sound therapies to soothe and align the mind.

Working with an Ayurvedic Practitioner

Ayurvedic practitioners take your health seriously and create a personalized plan for your well-being. However, they can only guide you—following through is up to you. If you don't take care of yourself, who will?

Ayurvedic medicine is about maintaining balance, preventing illness, and using natural methods to heal when needed. By embracing these practices, you can live a healthier, more balanced life.

How a Life Coach Can Help You

Life coaching is a powerful tool for personal and professional growth. Whether you're feeling stuck, facing challenges, or simply striving to reach your potential, a life coach can help you break through barriers, set clear goals, and take actionable steps to achieve them. Life coaches don't just focus on problems; they empower you to unlock your strengths, clarify your vision, and live a more fulfilling life.

How Can a Life Coach Help?

Life coaches provide guidance and support in many areas of life. They are not therapists or counselors; instead, they focus on the present and future, helping you move forward with purpose. Here are some ways a life coach can help:

- Goal Setting: Helping you define clear, realistic, and measurable goals.
- Accountability: Keeping you on track and motivated to achieve your objectives.
- Overcoming Blocks: Identifying and addressing obstacles, fears, or limiting beliefs that hold you back.
- Clarity: Offering an outside perspective to help you see situations more clearly.
- Personal Growth: Encouraging self-discovery and helping you grow into your best self.

Different Types of Life Coaches

There's a wide variety of life coaches, and chances are there's a specialist out there who can help with whatever issues or goals you're dealing with. Some of the most common types include:

- Career Coaches: Help you navigate job changes, improve workplace performance, or discover your ideal career path.
- Health and Wellness Coaches: Focus on improving physical health, managing stress, or creating healthier habits.
- Relationship Coaches: Assist with dating, communication, or building stronger relationships.
- Spiritual Coaches: Help you connect with your spiritual self or navigate life from a deeper, more purposeful perspective.
- Financial Coaches: Provide guidance on budgeting, saving, and achieving financial independence.
- Confidence Coaches: Work on self-esteem, assertiveness, and overcoming self-doubt.
- Life Transition Coaches: Support you through major life changes, such as divorce, retirement, or relocation.

- Performance Coaches: Help athletes, artists, or professionals improve their performance and mindset.
- Business Coaches: Guide entrepreneurs and business owners in growing their businesses or improving leadership skills.
- Creativity Coaches: Help writers, artists, or innovators overcome creative blocks and unlock their potential.

Whatever challenges or aspirations you have, there's likely a life coach who specializes in helping people like you.

Becoming a Life Coach

If you feel inspired to help others unlock their potential, becoming a life coach could be a rewarding path. Here's how you can get started:

Explore Your Interests: Think about the areas you're most passionate about, such as health, relationships, or career development. This can help you identify your niche.

Get Educated: While no formal education is required, completing a life coaching certification program can enhance your skills and credibility.

Practice Coaching: Start by offering coaching to friends, family, or volunteer clients to develop your skills and confidence.

Build a Business: Create a website, define your services, and start marketing your coaching practice. Social media, networking, and referrals can help you attract clients.

Continue Learning: Successful coaches invest in their own growth. Attend workshops, read books, and seek mentorship to keep improving.

Join a Community: Connect with other coaches through professional organizations or online groups to share experiences and resources.

Why Work with a Life Coach?

Working with a life coach is an investment in yourself. It's a way to gain clarity, focus, and support in achieving your dreams. Whether you're struggling to overcome obstacles or simply want to accelerate your growth, a life coach can provide the tools, encouragement, and accountability you need.

If you're curious about becoming a coach, it's a chance to turn your passion for helping others into a meaningful career. Life coaching isn't just about guiding others—it's also a journey of personal growth and transformation.

Throughout human history, cultures from every corner of the world have developed unique ways to heal, grow, and connect with the deeper currents of life. These practices, often referred to as "modalities," are gifts from our ancestors—each one shaped by the wisdom of its time and place. Yet, despite their differences, they all share a universal goal: to bring harmony to the mind, body, and spirit. This shared intention reminds us of the profound interconnectedness of all humanity.

In China, the ancient practice of acupuncture aligns the body's energy, or qi, by stimulating specific points to promote healing and balance. In India, Ayurveda, one of the oldest medical systems, teaches that health arises from harmony among the body, mind, and environment. Indigenous peoples across the Americas use ceremonial practices, such as sweat lodges and smudging, to cleanse the spirit and restore inner peace.

What's remarkable is how these modalities, developed in isolation across continents, reflect universal truths about the human experience. They show us that healing isn't just about addressing physical symptoms—it's about nurturing the whole person, connecting to the Earth, and finding alignment within and with others.

As we explore modalities like Reiki from Japan, reflexology rooted in ancient Egypt, or herbal wisdom from the Celtic traditions of Europe, we can see the beauty of inclusion. Each practice carries unique insights, yet they all point to a shared understanding: that the world's diverse paths to wellness are threads in the same universal tapestry.

In embracing these ancient teachings, we honor the idea that healing isn't limited to one culture or way of thinking. It's a collective gift from humanity's collective past—a reminder that, no matter where we come from, we all seek to live in balance and harmony. By learning from each other's wisdom, we can open ourselves to deeper connection, understanding, and a more profound sense of unity.

10 NATURAL ALTERNATIVE TOOLS

When I first started exploring natural remedies, I felt a deep connection to something ancient and profound. I was drawn to the idea that nature provides everything we need to heal—not just our bodies, but our minds and spirits too. It wasn't long before I realized that being an herbalist required more than knowledge of plants; it required tools, care, and a sense of respect for the Earth's gifts.

My herbal journey began with simple tools—a mortar and pestle, a few jars, and a good tea strainer. I loved the hands-on process of grinding herbs, inhaling their rich aromas, and watching as their healing properties transformed into teas, tinctures, or balms. Over time, I came to see my tools as more than just objects; they became partners in the art of healing.

Every jar I filled, every dropper I used, and every bundle of herbs I tied felt like an act of gratitude to the natural world. The process taught me patience, respect, and the beauty of working with my hands to create something that could help others.

Herbalism isn't just about mixing plants—it's about creating harmony. Whether you're crafting a remedy for a loved one or exploring the healing properties of a new herb, you're part of a tradition that stretches back through time, across cultures, and around the world. Your tools become your bridge to this ancient wisdom, connecting you to the plants, the Earth, and the people you aim to help.

As you assemble your herbalist tool kit, remember that it's more than a collection of items. It's a symbol of your commitment to healing naturally, honoring the balance of life, and embracing the endless possibilities found in nature's bounty. This journey is about more than tools and techniques—it's about building a relationship with the Earth and sharing its wisdom with others.

Your Herbalist Tool Kit

If you're thinking about becoming an herbalist, you'll need to assemble a tool kit with everything necessary to start creating natural remedies. Here's a detailed guide to help you get started and ensure your tools are ready for the job.

Essential Tools for an Herbalist

Filter

Filters are used to strain plant materials, leaving a clear liquid that's easy to consume. Avoid using metal strainers, as metal can change the chemical properties of herbs and create harmful metallic oxides.

Opt for natural, uncolored cotton or linen cloth, disposable coffee filters, or a plastic coffee cone filter. Always use clean, unused materials to avoid contamination.

Bamboo Tea Strainer

This is another useful tool, but keep in mind that finely ground herbs may pass through its holes. Use it with coarser herbs for better results.

Infuser

An infuser heats water and seals in steam to extract the best properties of herbs. A teapot works well, but it's important to avoid metal. Look for a pot with a tight lid, such as one glazed with enamel, to prevent steam from escaping.

Measuring Cups

Precise measurements are crucial for herbal preparations. Choose non-metallic measuring cups, and use the same tool consistently for accuracy. If you don't have a measuring cup, some herbalists use their palm as a guide in a pinch.

Additional Tools for Your Kit

First Aid Kit

Keep plenty of bandages and gauze on hand for minor injuries while working with herbs or gardening.

Small Bottles

Dark bottles are ideal for storing oils and tinctures, as they block sunlight that can degrade the contents. Always clean the bottles thoroughly before use.

Eye Droppers

Eye droppers are essential for measuring and dispensing liquids. Ensure the rubber tops are removable so they can be cleaned properly.

Glass Funnel

A funnel helps you transfer liquids into bottles without spills.

Hand Towel

Set aside a towel specifically for your tools. It should only be used for your herbal work to maintain cleanliness.

Shovel

A small shovel is helpful for gathering herbs from your garden or the wild.

Sharp Knife

Use a dedicated knife for cutting herbs and stems. It should be sharp enough to handle tough branches.

String

Use string to tie herb bundles together for drying.

Labels and Index Cards

Labels are a must for identifying what's in your jars and bottles. Write down the herb name and the date it was prepared. Use index cards to record recipes or experiments so you don't forget the ingredients.

The Mortar and Pestle: A Key Herbalist Tool

Once your herbs are harvested and dried, it's time to grind them. This releases the essential oils and healing properties trapped in the plant.

Material Matters:

Stone mortars are the best choice because they don't absorb moisture or scents. Wood mortars can retain oils from previous herbs, which may interfere with your current preparation.

Choose a mortar that is durable and can handle the pressure of grinding roots and seeds.

How to Use It:

Chop roots into smaller pieces to make grinding easier.

Grind herbs into a fine powder to maximize the release of their essential oils.

Enjoy the process—it's not just functional but also a sensory experience. The aroma of the herbs as you grind them is a reminder of the healing power you're preparing to share.

Storing Your Herbs Properly

Once your herbs are dried, you'll need to store them carefully to preserve their potency.

Sealed Containers

Use jars with tight-fitting lids to keep herbs fresh. Colored jars (blue, green, or brown) block sunlight, which can cause herbs to lose their effectiveness. Clear jars can be used if stored in a dark cupboard or cabinet.

Where to Find Jars

Look for jars at garage sales, thrift stores, or Goodwill. Family and friends might also help you find jars, or you can request them as gifts for birthdays or holidays.

Labeling and Dating

Always label jars with the name of the herb and the preparation date. This helps track potency and ensures you know what's inside.

Tips for Success

Keep Tools Separate: Only use your herbal tools for preparing herbs. This prevents cross-contamination and keeps your remedies pure.

Clean After Each Use: Wash your tools thoroughly after every use to avoid contaminating your next preparation.

Start Small: When blending herbs, work with small batches to reduce waste and learn as you go.

The Joy of Herbalism

As an herbalist, you'll discover the endless possibilities nature has to offer. Every herb holds healing potential, and the more you explore, the more you'll uncover. Your mortar and pestle, along with your carefully chosen tools, will help you transform plants into teas, tinctures, and remedies that can improve health and well-being.

Remember, herbalism is not just about tools—it's about love, patience, and learning. The world is your garden, and there are treasures waiting to be found. Take care of your tools, stay curious, and enjoy the journey of creating natural remedies.

The Art of Healing: A Journey with Nature

The wisdom of the old ways teaches that the Earth provides everything needed to nurture and heal. The practice of herbalism, rooted in ancient traditions, reflects a deep connection to nature's rhythms and an understanding of the balance between the human body and the natural world.

The Tools of Connection

In indigenous teachings, tools are not just objects but extensions of intention and care. Preparing natural remedies is a sacred act, and each tool—from the humble mortar and pestle to the jars that hold dried herbs—is part of a relationship with the plants and their healing properties. By respecting these tools and their purpose, we honor the gifts of the Earth.

Mindful Preparation

The process of creating herbal remedies mirrors the cycles of nature: planting, harvesting, and transforming. Every step requires patience and respect, reminding us to work in harmony with the land. The tools used, chosen with care and maintained with love, reflect this mindfulness, ensuring that the remedies we prepare carry the purity and strength of the plants themselves.

Learning from the Land

Herbalism is a journey of discovery. Each plant is a teacher, offering lessons not just in healing but in resilience, adaptability, and abundance. The tools of the herbalist become bridges, connecting the wisdom of the plants with the needs of the body and spirit.

Preservation and Gratitude

The old ways emphasize the importance of preserving the gifts of nature. Proper storage, careful labeling, and a respect for each plant's life cycle ensure that nothing is wasted. This practice fosters gratitude for the abundance around us and a commitment to care for the Earth so it may continue to provide.

Healing Beyond the Physical

Herbalism is more than the preparation of remedies; it is a reflection of the healer's connection to the natural world. Each herb carries not only physical healing properties but also the energy of the Earth, reinforcing the bond between human life and the cycles of nature.

As the elders teach, "To work with the plants is to work with the spirit of the Earth." By approaching herbalism with respect, curiosity, and love, we align ourselves with this ancient wisdom, carrying forward the healing traditions that have sustained humanity for generations. Let each remedy be a testament to the harmony between the healer and the land.

11 SOCIETAL IMPACT

As I look at the world around me, it's clear that society is at a crossroads. We're facing challenges on every front—economic instability, environmental destruction, social division, and now, global health crises. But with these challenges also comes an opportunity: a chance to rethink how we live, how we treat each other, and how we use the tools and resources at our disposal to create meaningful change.

For me, this chapter is about exploring the tools—both tangible and intangible—that can help us navigate these times. It's about understanding how ancient wisdom and modern innovations can work together to address the issues we face as individuals and as a collective. Whether it's learning from the past, embracing new ideas, or building connections across cultures and communities, I believe we have the ability to create a more balanced and equitable world.

But it starts with awareness. It starts with asking hard questions, challenging assumptions, and being open to new ways of thinking. This chapter is an invitation to look beyond the surface and consider the deeper systems and structures that shape our lives. It's about finding the tools to not only survive but thrive, in a way that honors the Earth, respects humanity, and leaves a better world for those who come after us. Let's explore this together.

Top Greed: How It Affects Us All

Have you ever thought about how everything on this planet is just trying to survive? From humans to animals, everyone works hard in their own way to get through each day. Humans go to work to feed their families, pay for a home, and provide clothes for their kids. Animals, on the other hand, search for food in the wild or eat the scraps we leave behind.

But both humans and animals are being harmed by the greed of a few. Little by little, our way of life is being destroyed. Yet, many people don't see it. We're distracted, arguing over small things, and missing the bigger picture.

Losing Our Freedom

People often say, "This is the land of the free." But how free are we when we're losing so much? Homes that families worked hard to pay off can be taken away if they can't afford property taxes. Even if your house is paid in full, you're never truly secure if taxes become unaffordable. And when that happens, no one seems to care about what happens to you.

Have you ever stopped to think:

- Who makes these rules?
- Who benefits from them?

It's not always clear. Banks seem to be one of the culprits, but they often ask for bailouts when they're struggling. So who is really in control? The government? Or someone else?

Powerful Families and Hidden Agendas

When I was younger, I heard about powerful, wealthy families who had a lot of influence over governments because of their money. At the time, I didn't think it mattered. It felt like something far away, unrelated to my life.

But now, as I've grown older and seen dramatic changes in the world, I realize how much these forces affect us. For example, there are cures for diseases like cancer that could save lives, but we don't hear about them. Why? Because sharing those cures would mean less money for powerful corporations and their partners in government. Greed keeps these solutions hidden from us.

The Federal Reserve and False Security

The Federal Reserve is one of the biggest scams in the system. It creates money, pumps it into the economy, and gives people a false sense of security. People start spending, taking on debt, and believing everything is fine—until the economy crashes. When that happens, people lose their jobs, homes, and businesses, yet they're still expected to pay back their debts. It's a vicious cycle that benefits the powerful while leaving ordinary people struggling.

Our Voices Are Being Silenced

We're told that in a democracy, everyone's voice matters. But does it? Many of the people we elect to represent us in Congress aren't listening to us. Instead, they're being influenced by companies and special interest groups that can afford to "buy" their votes. Ordinary people, who don't have the money to compete, are left unheard.

What Can We Do?

It's time to pay attention and ask tough questions:

Why are we fighting over small things while the powerful take away our freedom?

How can we hold those in power accountable for the greed and corruption that harm us all?

The truth is, greed at the top affects everyone. By staying informed and united, we can start to push back and demand a system that works for the many, not just the few.

Consequences of Greed

The wisdom of the old ways teaches that life thrives when harmony and balance guide our actions. Indigenous traditions from the champions of the first cultures remind us that greed disrupts this balance, creating suffering not only for humans but for all living beings. When a few prioritize personal gain over the well-being of the whole, the web of life is weakened, and the natural cycles that sustain us are threatened.

The Illusion of Ownership

In traditional teachings, the land, water, and sky are sacred and belong to no one. They are gifts to be shared and cared for, not commodities to be exploited. When greed takes hold, it fosters the illusion of ownership, leading to the hoarding of resources and the dispossession of those who depend on them. The ancestors warn that no one truly owns the Earth—our role is to protect and steward it for future generations.

The Interconnectedness of All Life

The Earth's balance relies on every being fulfilling its role. When humans overstep, taking more than needed or exploiting others, the balance is disrupted, leading to cycles of suffering. Primal knowledge teaches that what harms one part of the cultural weaving ultimately harms the whole. By ignoring this truth, we risk not only the health of the planet but our own survival.

The Cost of Distraction

Greed thrives in the shadows, taking advantage of division and distraction. When communities argue over small differences, they lose sight of the greater forces at play. The old ways call us to look beyond surface conflicts and unite against the deeper injustices that threaten the harmony of life.

Reclaiming Power Through Unity

The teachings of the ancestors remind us that true power lies in the collective. When people come together with shared purpose, they can challenge systems of greed and create a future rooted in equity and care. The key is remembering our connection to one another and the Earth, and using that connection to guide our actions.

A Path Forward

The old ways call for a return to balance, humility, and accountability. By prioritizing the well-being of the whole over individual gain, we can rebuild systems that honor the sacred interconnectedness of life. This begins with asking hard questions, seeking truth, and refusing to remain silent in the face of injustice.

As the elders teach, "The Earth provides for every need, but not for every greed." Let us walk with intention, restoring harmony to our communities and our planet, and ensuring a future where all beings can thrive.

Microchip or Not? Should I Get It?

Would you let someone put a microchip under your skin? It's a question I've asked a few people, and the answers are usually split. Some say yes, thinking it would be convenient, while others say no.

What's the Appeal?

Some people believe getting a microchip is a good idea. They say:

- You can pay for things just by waving your hand.
- In a medical emergency, the chip can be scanned to provide your health information instantly.

It might sound helpful, but there's more to think about.

A Way to Control?

The government and corporations could use this technology to control people. History shows us that many good inventions start with good intentions but often end up being misused.

At first, the microchip might seem like a personal choice. It's marketed as:

- Convenient
- Easy to use
- Great for safety

But who benefits the most? Is it really for you—or for those in power?

How Do Microchips Work?

There are different kinds of microchips:

Some are injected under your skin, like a tiny tattoo.

Others might come with a vaccine and can only be scanned using special devices, like smartphones.

Many people have tried these chips and say it makes their lives easier. Some companies are even thinking about making them mandatory for employees.

Right now, you have a choice to say no. But what happens if it becomes required? What if you can't work, shop, or pay for anything without one? That's where control begins—what starts as a choice could become a demand.

The Risks

Have you thought about how a microchip might affect your health? Here are some of the risks:

- Cancer and Tumors: Studies have shown that microchips can cause cancerous growths or tumors in animals and possibly in humans.
- Infections: The injection site can swell, get infected, or ooze pus.
- Chip Movement: Once inside your body, the chip can move, making it hard to find in an emergency.
- Interference with Medical Devices: MRI machines, defibrillators, and other devices may not work properly if you have a microchip.

These are serious concerns, but companies still push the technology as if it's completely safe.

Is It Worth the Risk?

Before getting a microchip, ask yourself:

- Is this really worth the risk to my health?
- Could this technology be used to control me in the future?

Sure, it might make opening a door or changing the TV channel easier. But is convenience worth the long-term effects on your health and freedom?

The Bigger Picture

Technology can make life easier, but it often comes with side effects that aren't worth the price. Some risks take years to show up, and by then, it might be too late.

In the end, I'd rather stay healthy and in control of my life than regret a decision that could change everything. Always think carefully before putting your health and freedom on the line.

Navigating the Path of Technology

The wisdom of the ancestors teaches us to walk carefully with new tools, to honor the gifts of innovation while remaining vigilant about their impact. Indigenous traditions from the inheritors of the timeless legacy remind us that every choice carries consequences, both seen and unseen. When considering powerful technologies, the old ways encourage reflection, balance, and a deep understanding of the connection between our bodies, our freedoms, and the Earth.

Tools as Allies, Not Masters

In traditional teachings, tools are seen as extensions of human intent—servants of purpose, not masters of the soul. The ancestors warn against giving away control to something outside ourselves. When tools, no matter how advanced, begin to dictate how we live or limit our freedoms, they risk disrupting the balance that sustains harmony in life.

The Wisdom of Choice

Choice is a sacred gift, one that must be exercised with awareness and foresight. The old ways teach that true freedom lies in the ability to question, to listen deeply, and to act in alignment with the greater good. Before embracing something new, the question must be asked: Does this tool serve me, or does it serve those who seek to control me?

The Balance of Convenience and Consequence

Convenience is tempting, but it often comes with hidden costs. The Earth teaches us that every shortcut has its price—whether in health, freedom, or spiritual well-being. By observing the cycles of nature, the old ways remind us that nothing comes without responsibility. Each step forward must be weighed against what might be lost.

Guarding the Sacred

The body, in native wisdom, is a sacred vessel—connected to the land, the spirit, and the community. Altering or embedding foreign objects into the body is not a decision to be made lightly. It requires careful consideration of the potential risks to health and the possible loss of autonomy.

A Call to Reflection

The teachings of the old ways encourage us to pause, to reflect, and to seek wisdom before moving forward. Decisions made in haste, without thought for the long-term impact, can lead to regret. The Earth and its cycles remind us to move slowly and deliberately, honoring the interconnectedness of all life.

Walking the Middle Path

Technology is not inherently harmful; it is how we use it that determines its impact. The ancestors teach that balance is key—embracing progress while remaining grounded in timeless truths. By keeping our hearts open and our minds clear, we can navigate the challenges of modern life without losing sight of what truly matters.

As the elders say, "The greatest tool you will ever have is your own wisdom." Let us honor this wisdom, making choices that preserve our health, our freedoms, and our connection to the Earth and one another.

Prejudice: Are We Born This Way?

Have you ever wondered why some people are prejudiced? Why do they treat others so poorly just because of how they look or speak? What could have happened to make one person hate an entire group of people?

Sadly, prejudice is all around us. Many people treat others as though they are less than human—sometimes worse than animals. At least animals are often treated with kindness, while some people treat others with cruelty and disrespect.

Slavery: A Dark Part of History

From a young age, we learn in history books about slavery and how people were once considered valuable based on how many slaves they owned. This happened all over the world and, unfortunately, still exists today, though it goes by different names.

One of the most common forms today is human trafficking.

- Sex Trafficking: Young people are taken and sold into the sex trade.
- Child Labor: Children are forced to work long hours for little or no pay.
- Unfair Wages: Even adults in some jobs are not paid fairly for their hard work.

Many workers are treated poorly, especially by owners of large companies. Some business owners act as if their employees are beneath them, forgetting that without workers, their companies wouldn't exist.

Kindness Builds a Stronger Workforce

How you treat people says a lot about you. If you are fair, kind, and respectful to everyone—no matter their position—you create an amazing work environment.

Employees thrive when they feel appreciated.

A simple compliment can boost morale and productivity.

Unfortunately, some managers abuse their power. They treat employees unfairly, threaten their jobs, or act superior. Being in a higher position doesn't give anyone the right to mistreat others.

Prejudice Starts Early

Prejudice isn't something we are born with—it's something we are taught. Some people grow up hearing harmful ideas, like:

People who don't look like us are bad.

People who speak a different language are talking about us behind our backs.

Teaching children these ideas only spreads ignorance and hate. It's unfair and harmful to judge an entire group of people because of the actions of a few.

Judging an Entire Group

One bad person doesn't define an entire race, culture, or group. Every community has good and bad people. Prejudice assumes that everyone in a group is the same, but that simply isn't true. Many people work hard to fight against the wrongs done by others in their own communities.

We Can Make a Difference

We have the power to create a better world. Instead of only coming together during disasters, we should work together during times of peace. By treating others with kindness and respect, we can break the cycle of prejudice.

Are We Born Prejudiced?

So, are we born prejudiced—or are we taught to be? Prejudice isn't something that comes naturally. It's something learned through words, actions, and examples set by others. But just as prejudice can be taught, kindness and acceptance can be taught too. It's up to us to choose what kind of world we want to live in.

Breaking the Cycle of Separation

The teachings of the ancestors remind us that all life is connected, woven together like the threads of a sacred blanket. To harm one thread is to weaken the whole, and to separate ourselves from others is to deny the truth of our shared humanity. Prejudice, with its roots in fear and ignorance, is not part of our natural state but something learned, something that can be unlearned.

The Illusion of Division

Cultural wisdom teaches that the Earth does not see borders, races, or languages. It provides for all without discrimination, nourishing each being equally. Prejudice arises when we forget this truth, when we begin to see differences as barriers rather than blessings. The ancestors knew that diversity in nature strengthens the whole; the same is true for humanity.

Lessons from the Circle

In the sacred circle, all are equal—no one sits higher, and no one sits lower. This is a reflection of the balance and harmony that the old ways strive to maintain. Judging others disrupts this balance, creating a world of "us" and "them," where none can thrive. Instead, the circle calls for understanding, for seeing each being as a vital part of the whole.

Taught, Not Born

The wisdom of the old ways acknowledges that fear of the unfamiliar is often passed down, not inherent. Children are like blank pages, and the stories written on their hearts shape their worldview. When they are taught respect, kindness, and the value of all life, they grow into adults who honor the sacred connections between all beings.

Healing Through Unity

Prejudice can be unlearned, just as harmony can be restored to the land after it is scarred. The path forward requires patience, humility, and a willingness to listen deeply—to others, to the Earth, and to the stories of those who have suffered. By coming together, we can mend the divisions that weaken us and build a future rooted in mutual respect.

A Choice for the Future

The ancestors remind us that we have the power to choose. Just as seeds grow into trees, our actions today shape the world of tomorrow. By choosing kindness over judgment and unity over division, we plant seeds of harmony that will bear fruit for generations to come.

As the elders say, "The heart that sees no difference sees the truth." Let us walk with open hearts, honoring the shared humanity that connects us all, and teaching future generations the wisdom of love and understanding.

Celebrate or Confiscate Cell Phones?

Have you ever heard someone say, "Back in my day, we didn't have cell phones"? It's true—things were very different before smartphones came along. Kids used to play outside until it got dark. We didn't need to be called back home; we just knew when it was time.

Back then, technology didn't keep us indoors. Neighborhood kids would get together to:

- Play ball
- Ride bikes
- Get into a little harmless mischief

If there was a disagreement, it might lead to a fistfight—but that was usually off school grounds. At school, getting caught fighting meant a trip to the principal's office for a paddling. There were no school shootings or widespread violence like we hear about today.

The Role of Technology Today

Times have changed. Now, kids often stay inside playing games on:

- PlayStations
- X-Boxes
- Computers
- Cell Phones

When we were kids, the only phone we had was a landline. It hung on the wall or sat on a table, and it didn't have caller ID or voicemail. If you missed a call, the person just had to call back. We even had a phone number to call just to find out the time!

Phones back then were simple, but they didn't distract us from life the way today's phones can.

The Good Side of Cell Phones

There's no denying that modern cell phones have made life easier in some ways. They're useful for:

- Emergencies: You can call for help from almost anywhere.
- Everyday tasks: Phones act as a camera, clock, calendar, and calculator all in one.
- Staying connected: They let us communicate with people around the world instantly.

The Downside of Cell Phones

While phones have made life more convenient, they've also created new problems.

Strangers Become Closer, Families Grow Apart

Phones make it easy to connect with people across the globe, but sometimes they make us distant from the people we love most.

Kids Without Phones Are Left Out

In the past, kids could use a family landline to call for help or talk to someone they trusted. Now, many kids without their own phone have no way to reach out.

Parents Distracted by Phones

Too often, parents are glued to their screens, ignoring their kids. There have been real-life situations where this has led to dangerous moments:

A father at the park was so focused on his phone that he didn't notice someone trying to walk off with his child. A bystander had to intervene and warn him to pay attention.

A couple with a baby carriage was too distracted by their phones to notice a car backing out and nearly hitting their child. A stranger saved the baby by pushing the carriage out of the way and smashing the parents' phones in frustration.

Should We Celebrate or Confiscate Cell Phones?

Cell phones are powerful tools, but they come with risks. They can help us in emergencies and make life easier in many ways. Yet, they also take us away from what matters most—our families, our safety, and our real-life connections.

So, what do you think? Should we celebrate the convenience of cell phones or confiscate them to focus on what really matters? The choice is ours to make.

The Balance Between Connection and Distraction

In the wisdom of the ancestors, life was guided by simplicity, connection, and purpose. Tools, whether crafted by hand or borrowed from nature, were always meant to serve life—not control it. Indigenous teachings from the pioneers of ancestral wisdom remind us to walk in balance, embracing what is useful while remaining grounded in what is real.

The Power of Tools

The old ways teach that tools, whether they be ancient stones or modern devices, are neither good nor bad. They carry the intention of their user. A tool that fosters connection, enhances safety, or makes life easier is a gift when used with mindfulness. But when a tool becomes a distraction, pulling us away from what matters most, it loses its purpose and risks becoming a burden.

The Gift of Presence

True connection is not found in screens or distant voices but in the presence of shared moments. Indigenous cultures emphasize the importance of being fully present—with the land, with the community, and with oneself. To live well is to give your full attention to those around you, to listen deeply, and to honor the sacredness of time spent together.

Lessons from the Past

There was a time when connection meant gathering under the stars, telling stories by the fire, or sharing laughter in the open air. These moments were not interrupted by distractions but enriched by the simplicity of human connection. The ancestors remind us that these moments are still available to us—if we are willing to put aside what pulls us away.

Finding Balance in Modern Life

The teachings of the old ways do not ask us to reject progress but to integrate it thoughtfully. Just as fire must be tended to avoid burning the forest, modern tools like cell phones must be used with care to avoid consuming our attention and energy. Balance can be found by using these tools as aids rather than allowing them to dominate our lives.

Returning to What Matters

The Earth calls us back to the wisdom of presence. Whether walking in nature, sitting with family, or simply observing the world around us, we are reminded that the truest connections are those we nurture in real time. When we put down distractions, we open ourselves to the beauty and depth of life.

A Path Forward

The ancestors teach that the choice is always ours. We can celebrate the gifts of technology while remaining mindful of its influence. By setting boundaries, honoring moments of presence, and prioritizing human connection, we can ensure that our tools serve us, not the other way around.

In the words of the elders: "Be where your feet are. The world moves at its own rhythm—walk with it, not apart from it." Let us embrace the gifts of modern life while staying rooted in the timeless wisdom of presence and connection.

The Food Chain: Why Every Creature Matters

Every creature on Earth has a purpose, from the smallest to the largest. Each one plays an important role in keeping the planet healthy and balanced.

Take the earthworm, for example. It lives underground, creating natural fertilizer that helps plants grow. Bees collect nectar from flowers for food, and in the process, they spread pollen to help fruits and seeds grow. Even spiders, which some people fear, help keep unwanted insects out of gardens. Did you know a spider can eat 10% of its body weight in a single day? That's a lot of pests being controlled!

How Animals Depend on Each Other

Every animal helps keep other animals in check. They all depend on one another to survive. Without this balance, life on Earth would fall apart.

Humans are at the top of the food chain, and we eat more than any other creature. Unlike a spider, we sometimes try to eat as much as our weight in food! Unfortunately, we are also the most wasteful.

Food Waste and Overconsumption

We throw away perfectly good food just because it doesn't look right—maybe it's the wrong shape or color. Instead of feeding the hungry, this food is often left to rot. In the past, people used every part of an animal, from the head to the hooves. Now, much of it is wasted.

Some people even hunt animals like deer and elk for sport rather than food. While every creature works hard to survive, humans often take more than we need.

The Overarching Vision

Every living thing, from land animals to sea creatures, needs our help. Without them, life on Earth wouldn't survive. Think about our oceans, where animals like fish, turtles, and seals face threats from pollution and abandoned fishing nets. These nets trap animals, causing them to drown or lose limbs.

What Can We Do?

It's up to us to make a change. Here's how we can start:

- Protect Wildlife: Care for land and sea creatures by reducing waste and pollution.

- Stop Food Waste: Use what you have and share extra food with those in need.
- Recycle: Pick up trash and recycle, especially near oceans and rivers.

Why It Matters

Every action we take helps protect life on Earth. By saving animals and plants, we also help ourselves. Imagine a world without these creatures—it would be a tragedy for all of us.

Let's think positively and work together to protect our planet. Even small steps, like picking up a piece of trash or making smarter food choices, can make a big difference. Remember, every life saved is a step toward saving our own.

A Lesson from the Earth

In the world that we live in, every being plays a role, from the smallest creature to the most powerful. The teachings of native peoples from the bearers of the ancient ways remind us that all life is interconnected. No creature exists in isolation; each contributes to the delicate balance that sustains the Earth.

The Sacred Circle of Life

The old ways speak of a great circle, where every life is connected, each link essential. From the creatures of the soil to those of the sky and sea, all contribute to the health of the planet. When one part of the circle is broken—through neglect or overconsumption—the balance begins to falter, affecting all who depend on it.

Lessons from the Smallest Teachers

Even the humblest beings, such as those who dwell beneath the soil or in the water, offer profound lessons. They are caretakers of the land, working tirelessly to nurture growth and renewal. To overlook their importance is to forget the wisdom of nature, which shows us that strength lies not in size but in purpose.

Responsibility at the Top

Humanity, as stewards of this world, bears the greatest responsibility. Elder wisdom teaches that leadership is not about domination but about care and respect for all beings. The privilege of abundance calls for gratitude, and the ability to take must be balanced with the willingness to give back.

Waste as a Wound

The old ways warn against waste, which dishonors the gifts of the Earth. Every part of what is taken should be used, and nothing discarded without purpose. When wastefulness becomes a habit, it erodes not only the land but also the spirit, separating us from the harmony that sustains life.

A Path to Renewal

The teachings of the ancestors show us that even small actions can restore balance. Caring for the land, respecting its creatures, and taking only what is needed can bring healing to the Earth. By learning from the wisdom of the circle, we can ensure that life continues to thrive for generations to come.

Walking in Balance

The Earth offers countless reminders that we are not separate from nature—we are a part of it. Each step we take on this path is an opportunity to honor the interconnectedness of life. As the elders teach, when we walk in balance with the world around us, we create a future where all beings can flourish.

Let us remember that every creature matters, every action counts, and every life is sacred. Together, we can protect the circle of life, ensuring its strength for those who will follow.

Man's Greed

Our planet is home to so many beautiful animals, as well as some that aren't as cute or friendly. The Earth itself is full of amazing places, some breathtaking and others intimidating. Every creature has its place, from the freezing tundras to scorching deserts. They survive in ways that show incredible adaptability and strength.

But as humans expand and take over more land, animals are being forced into smaller, crowded spaces. Forests and trees are being cut down daily, leaving many creatures without food or shelter. How can we think this is okay? Taking away their homes and food makes it nearly impossible for them to survive.

The Problem with Greed

The greed of a few humans is responsible for much of this destruction. Not all people are to blame, but those with power and money often prioritize profits over the well-being of animals, plants, or even other people. They destroy without caring about the lives they harm.

The Earth has an amazing ability to heal itself, just like our bodies do when we're hurt or sick. But even Earth needs help sometimes. Pollution in the air, contamination in the food we eat, and chemicals in the water we drink are taking a toll. If we don't make changes soon, both humans and animals may not survive for much longer.

The Cost of Modern Life

Diseases are becoming more common, and they affect not just people but pets too. Despite all the advances in technology, we're not getting healthier. There's still no cure for cancer or diabetes, and instead of focusing on lasting solutions, companies race to create pills that promise to make us feel young again.

But the answers we need might already be here, right in nature. The plants that grow around us hold so much healing potential. We just need to take the time to learn how to use them for our benefit.

A Wake-Up Call

It's time to stop and really look at the world around us. We already have what we need to live healthier, better lives. Let's not ignore the gifts of the Earth—or God's plan for us.

Technology has made life easier in so many ways, but we've become ungrateful. We complain about things that would have amazed our ancestors. They would see us as spoiled for not appreciating the conveniences we have today. They would marvel at the inventions that save time and make hard work easier, allowing us to spend more time with loved ones.

What Can We Do?

We need to shift our focus. Instead of taking more from the planet, we should work to protect it. Let's appreciate the resources we have and use them wisely. By doing so, we can create a better future—not just for ourselves, but for all the creatures we share this Earth with.

What's Going On? How Could It Be?

Common sense seems to be disappearing in today's world. Things that should be easy to understand often feel confusing, like we're being shown an illusion instead of reality. How can that happen?

We're constantly told things that seem true at first glance. But if you take the time to investigate, you often find they're not true at all. It's like someone is pulling the wool over your eyes, hoping you won't question it.

The saying, "Don't believe everything you hear or read," is more important now than ever. As I've gotten older, I've realized this more and more. Sometimes what I learn is disappointing, but it's also freeing. Knowing the truth means I'm not following blindly. I'm still learning and trying to understand the bigger picture.

How Do We Make a Change?

What will it take to make a real change in the world? It feels like we're more divided than ever. Instead of working together, we blame each other, pointing fingers at different races or groups. When will it stop?

The pandemic has only made things worse. We've been told to stay home, avoid socializing, and keep our distance from family and friends. This has left us feeling isolated and more divided than ever.

A Time of Uncertainty

Right now, life feels like a yo-yo. One moment things are getting better, and the next, we're right back where we started. It's like being stuck in a loop, going in circles, and nothing ever truly changes.

It's frustrating, but it also shows us that waiting for change isn't enough. We need to take action together.

When We Come Together

History shows that during times of tragedy, people often unite. When disaster strikes, we forget about differences like race, color, or language and work side by side to save lives. In those moments, we realize how much we can achieve when we help each other.

But why do we wait for tragedy to bring us together? Why not make unity a way of life? When we work together, we accomplish so much more, and the burden becomes lighter for everyone.

Building a United Future

The truth is, we don't have to wait for something bad to happen to come together. We can choose to be united now—before the next crisis. By supporting one another and working as a team, we can face anything that comes our way.

It's time to stop dividing ourselves and start thinking as one nation, united in every way. Together, we can create a stronger, better future for everyone. Let's not wait for another tragedy to show us what we're capable of. Let's start today.

Mankind's Consequences

Isn't it strange that in 2020, with all the advanced technology we have around the world, we still couldn't stop an epidemic from spreading? We couldn't even find a cure—or could we? The government isn't always honest about what it knows. It often hides things and creates stories to cover its tracks. This has happened many times throughout history.

The Hidden Inventions

I remember reading about a man who invented a car that could run on water. He said it would keep the air clean and save money because it didn't need gasoline. I even saw a picture of the prototype. But then, the story disappeared. Years later, I learned the inventor had been killed, and all his paperwork and the car itself had vanished.

There was another inventor who created a generator that could produce electricity on its own. It could have been affordable for everyone to have at home. But again, his work was destroyed, and nothing more was heard about it.

Why would these inventions disappear? Think about who would lose money if these ideas became reality. Companies that profit from gas, oil, and electricity would have been put out of business.

The Power of Greed

It's not just about inventions. Big pharmaceutical companies often fight against natural cures. How many times have you heard of someone finding a natural remedy only to be called a "quack" and ridiculed? These companies have a lot of money and power, and they use it to protect their profits.

All it takes is finding the right person in Congress who is willing to be bought. Sadly, there are many weak links in Congress and even in the White House. Promises are made to the people, but once elected, those promises are broken or forgotten.

The Bigger Picture

The real problem is greed. People with power only care about making money, no matter who or what gets hurt. They forget that humans share this planet with other living creatures. The destruction of land, animals, and even human lives doesn't matter to them as long as they make a profit.

A Call for Change

If we want a better future, we need leaders who can work together to make real changes—not just for humans, but for all living things. We need to stop ignoring the consequences of our actions. The planet, and everything on it, depends on us choosing responsibility over greed.

Let's not wait until it's too late to start caring about the world we live in. Every decision we make today shapes the future for all living creatures. It's time to think beyond profit and focus on what truly matters.

The Teachings of the Earth

In the stories of the land, passed down through generations, lies a truth that echoes across time: the Earth provides, but it also demands respect. Ancient traditions from the stewards of ancestral homelands remind us that all life is interconnected, and to harm one part of this web is to harm the whole.

The Balance of Giving and Taking

The old ways teach that nature thrives when there is harmony between giving and taking. To take more than needed, to destroy without thought, is to upset the balance that sustains all life. When greed drives actions, it leaves scars on the land, the animals, and even the human spirit. Yet, when respect and gratitude guide us, the Earth flourishes, providing enough for all.

The Power of Unity

The wisdom of the ancestors reminds us that division weakens, while unity strengthens. Times of hardship have shown that when humans come together, they can achieve remarkable things. But why wait for crisis to unite? By embracing shared purpose and mutual care now, we can heal not just the land, but also our communities.

The Gifts of Nature

The Earth is rich with resources, but these are not just for human consumption—they are part of a sacred cycle that supports all life. Plants hold the keys to health and healing; animals are teachers of resilience and adaptability. Native traditions teach that these gifts are to be used wisely, with reverence and an eye to the future, ensuring they endure for generations to come.

The Consequences of Greed

The lessons of the past warn against unchecked greed. When short-term profits are placed above long-term well-being, everyone suffers. The Earth begins to falter, animals disappear, and even human health deteriorates. The ancestors knew that wealth lies not in possessions but in the harmony of a thriving, balanced world.

Reclaiming Responsibility

The path forward calls for a return to responsibility and humility. By listening to the Earth, learning from its cycles, and respecting its limits, we honor the wisdom of those who came before us. This is not a call to abandon progress, but to redefine it—progress that aligns with the rhythms of nature and the needs of all life.

A Vision of Hope

The old ways teach that even when the Earth is wounded, it holds the power to heal. With care, patience, and cooperation, humanity can play a role in this healing. By planting seeds of respect and nurturing them with actions of compassion and unity, we can restore balance and create a future where all life thrives together.

Let us walk gently, remembering that the Earth is not just our home, but a sacred gift entrusted to us. As the elders say, "The land is not ours to own—it is ours to protect."

The Pandemic Outbreak

The COVID-19 pandemic has affected so many lives. People who've had the virus often describe feeling scared, unsure if they'd make it through. Symptoms can appear suddenly, and for some, it becomes a matter of life or death.

The more people survive this virus, the more we learn about how to help others cope and recover. Even mild cases can take a turn for the worse after three or four days. If you experience persistent chest pain, dizziness, or confusion—or if your lips start to turn blue—it's time to go to the hospital.

Helpful Tips for Coping with COVID-19

Ease Breathing: Use a humidifier to relieve chest tightness and reduce coughing.

Sleep on Your Stomach: Many people find it helps with symptoms. Sleeping on your side is a good alternative if stomach sleeping isn't comfortable.

Stay Active: Movement is important to keep your lungs clear. Even if you don't feel like getting out of bed, small movements can help.

Open a window for fresh air, and if you feel up to it, turn on some music and move gently—just don't overdo it.

Mental Health Matters

Being sick can make you feel stressed or depressed, but staying positive is important for recovery.

Talk to your doctor, friends, or family if you're feeling down.
Think of a happy memory and focus on it to boost your mood.
Even small steps can make a big difference in how you feel emotionally.

How Long Does Recovery Take?

Recovery times vary. Some people feel better in a few weeks, while others experience lingering symptoms for months. Unfortunately, it's possible to get COVID-19 again, and some report being sicker the second time. Scientists are still studying why this happens and how different strains of the virus affect people.

There's also uncertainty about how well vaccines protect against new strains. Will COVID-19 vaccinations become like the flu shot, needing updates for different strains? These are questions we're still seeking answers to.

Steps to Protect Yourself and Others

Wear a mask.
Keep 6 feet apart.
Wash your hands frequently.

Taking these precautions isn't a sign of weakness—it's a sign of respect for others. Those who think otherwise are missing the bigger picture.

Recovering from COVID-19

If you've had COVID-19, here are tips to help you recover:

Stay Active: Walk and stretch, but don't overdo it. Move during TV commercials or take short walks around the house.

Keep Moving: Light activity helps clear your lungs and keeps your body strong.

Sleep Smart: Sleep on your stomach or side to make breathing easier.

The Role of Natural Remedies

Doctors often recommend pharmaceutical medications, but some people prefer natural remedies. It's true that herbs have helped many people for centuries, and the body often responds well to them.

That said, it's important to use herbs safely. Taking too much can lead to harmful effects, like an overactive immune response called a cytokine storm. Always follow proper dosing and consult with a healthcare provider.

A Balanced Approach

While natural remedies can help, modern medicine is also important, especially for surgeries or emergencies like setting a broken bone. Both natural and medical approaches have their place in healing.

Stay Positive and Safe

Your mindset matters. Staying positive and following precautions—like wearing a mask, washing your hands, and keeping your distance—can make a big difference.

Remember, we've faced challenges as a nation before, and we can get through this too. Together, with respect and care for one another, we'll overcome the difficulties of this pandemic.

12 SEASONS CHANGE

I've always found the changing of the seasons to be magical. Each one has its own beauty, its own rhythm, and its own lessons to teach. Summer invites us to bask in abundance and energy, while autumn dazzles us with color and reminds us to prepare for what lies ahead. Winter slows everything down, urging us to rest and reflect, and then spring breathes new life into the world, bringing hope and renewal.

As I've grown older, I've realized how much the seasons mirror our own lives. There are times of growth, times of change, and times to simply be still and take it all in. Nature has a way of guiding us, showing us what we need if we take the time to listen.

This chapter is a celebration of the seasons and the lessons they offer. It's also a reminder of the sacred connection we share with the Earth. By appreciating and protecting the natural world, we honor its rhythms and ensure its beauty for generations to come. Let's explore how the seasons shape not just the world around us, but the lives we live within it.

The Four Seasons

Our planet has blessed us with the beauty of four seasons, each offering something special. From the warmth of summer to the stillness of winter, nature gives us so much to enjoy and appreciate.

Summer: A Season of Abundance

Summer is a time of life and joy. The birds sing, children run and laugh, and music seems to fill the air. While some people soak in the heat of the day, others dream of cooling off on a block of ice.

It's also the season when gardens overflow with fresh fruits and vegetables. For those who've worked hard in their gardens, summer is the reward. They harvest their crops, storing some in cellars, canning others, and sharing the rest with family and friends.

Autumn: A Time of Color and Change

Autumn is a breathtaking season, full of bright reds, yellows, oranges, and greens. The trees begin to shed their leaves, transforming the landscape into a colorful masterpiece.

As the days grow shorter and the sun's warmth fades, animals prepare for winter. Some gather food, while others eat as much as they can to build up fat for the colder months. Their coats grow thicker, and some even change color to blend in with the season.

Winter: A Season of Stillness

Winter brings cold temperatures and snow. In the past, survival depended on how well you prepared during summer and autumn. Today, there's more help available, but winter can still be harsh.

Snowfall is beautiful, soft, and silent, but it can also be dangerous. Without proper shelter, winter's cold can be deadly. However, for those who are prepared, winter offers its own kind of fun:

- Snowball fights (until someone gets hurt!)
- Building snowmen
- Making snow angels
- Constructing igloos

Despite its challenges, winter has its charm.

Spring: A Time of Renewal

Spring is when life begins to return. The days are still chilly, as if winter and spring are locked in a tug-of-war. Eventually, winter gives way, and spring brings new beginnings.

You'll see flowers pushing through the ground, baby animals being born, and trees budding. The warmth of the sun starts to return, waking the Earth from its slumber. It's a season of hope, a sign of the life and beauty to come.

A Reminder to Protect Our Planet

The Earth gives us so much—season after season, year after year. But as humans, we often take without giving back. Greed has led to the destruction of land and the creatures that call it home.

If we want to continue enjoying the beauty of the seasons, we must take care of our planet. Let's not forget the gifts nature provides and do our part to preserve them for future generations.

Listening to Nature

In our busy lives, we often forget to stop and notice the world around us. We rarely take time to sit quietly, relax, and enjoy the sounds of nature. Life feels like it's always on fast forward, and when we do sit down, what's the first thing we grab?

The remote control. The TV. Or the number one distraction—the phone!

Here's a joke:

Two crows are sitting on a phone line. One looks at a scarecrow below and says, "How do you know it's not human?" The other crow replies, "Because it's not looking at its phone!"

The Problem with Distractions

We're so attached to our devices that we sometimes put ourselves and others in danger. For example, people on their phones while driving might run a red light or stop sign. I've had a few close calls myself because of distracted drivers. If not for guardian angels, I might not be here to share this today.

We've become so focused on rushing through life that we don't stop to appreciate simple things like the smell of flowers, a walk in nature, or sitting on a porch to listen to birds or rain.

Finding Time to Relax

If you can't hear nature's sounds where you live, you can find them online. Search for sounds like:

- Ocean waves
- Flowing creeks
- Rainfall
- Soft music

If you have kids and find it hard to get quiet time, involve them! When my boys were little, I'd take them for walks in nature. At first, they'd complain and want to be carried. But with a few breaks to rest, they'd get through it. After dinner, a bath, and bedtime, my relaxing time would finally begin.

The Challenge with Technology and Kids

It's easy to let the TV or devices babysit our kids, but over time, this becomes a problem. They get so used to staying indoors that it becomes nearly impossible to get them outside.

Kids today are some of the least active and unhealthiest in history. They're spoiled by today's technology and miss out on the joys of playing outside.

Back in the Day

When I was a kid, as soon as breakfast was done, we were sent outside. We couldn't come back in until lunch—and then we were back outside again!

We didn't come inside for water; we drank from the garden hose. We played in the mud, got into harmless mischief, and had so much fun.

Reconnecting with Nature

It's time to put down our phones and reconnect with Mother Nature. Take a walk, sit outside, or just listen to the world around you. Teach your kids to enjoy the simple joys of being outdoors. Nature has so much to offer—don't let distractions make you miss it!

Dream About Enjoying a Natural Summer

Even though it's still winter—when the plants are dormant, the trees are bare, and the weather is rainy or snowy—it's the perfect time to start daydreaming about summer.

Picture This…

Have you ever visited a home with a beautiful yard and garden? Imagine sitting there on a warm summer day, a tall glass of iced tea in your hand. The sun warms your skin as you relax, watching nature all around you.

Bees buzz from one blossom to the next, carefully tending to each flower. Butterflies float by gracefully, their wings moving softly in the breeze. Birds sing their cheerful songs, splashing playfully in a birdbath.

A hummingbird zips past like it's late for an important meeting, only to stop and rest on a gorgeous plant, its tiny wings pausing for just a moment. The variety of plants in the garden not only brings beauty but also attracts birds, which help keep pesky bugs in check.

The Busy Life of Plants and Bugs

So much action happens around the plants. Some bugs are good, and some are bad. The key is knowing how to protect your garden by getting rid of harmful pests while keeping the helpful ones around.

That's why it's important to learn about plants that naturally protect your garden. Some plants are disliked by certain bugs because of their smell or taste, making them perfect for keeping pests away.

Plants That Protect Your Garden

Here are a few amazing plants that can naturally repel pests:

- Basil: Keeps flies and mosquitoes away.
- Chrysanthemums: Repels roaches, ants, and lice.
- Cilantro: Protects against spider mites.
- Mexican Marigold: Keeps insects and rabbits at bay.
- Narcissus: Repels gophers and rabbits.
- Russian Sage: Deters wasps.
- Spearmint: Drives away ants, moths, and rodents.

These plants don't just repel pests—they're also herbs that can heal the body and beautify your garden. Calling them "weeds" couldn't be more wrong. They're part of nature's way of helping us and the planet.

Plants: Earth's Helpers

Plants do more than add beauty to our gardens. They clean the air we breathe, making life better for everyone, especially those with breathing issues. Without plants, the air would be much worse, and life would be harder.

So, take time to appreciate your garden. Listen to the birds, watch the butterflies, and breathe in the fresh, fragrant air. Enjoy the vibrant colors and the peacefulness of nature.

A Warm Daydream for a Cold Season

Yes, it's still winter. The trees may be bare, and the wind may be chilly, but for a moment, you let your imagination take you to a warm, sunny garden. I know I did, and I hope you enjoyed the summer visions too.

The Circle of Seasons

In the rhythms of the Earth, the four seasons speak of balance, transformation, and renewal. Original cultures from the eternal spirits of the Earth teach us that each season holds a unique role in the sacred cycle of life. They remind us to honor these transitions, to live in harmony with nature, and to embrace the lessons each season offers.

The Gifts of Abundance and Preparation

The warm seasons teach us gratitude and stewardship. The Earth, abundant and generous, provides nourishment, growth, and beauty. Yet, the old ways remind us that abundance calls for responsibility. Just as our ancestors prepared during times of plenty, we too are asked to consider the future, taking only what is needed and offering thanks for what we receive.

The Wisdom of Change

As the Earth turns, the vibrant colors of transition reflect the impermanence of life. Leaves fall, days shorten, and creatures prepare for stillness. These moments of change teach patience, adaptability, and the necessity of letting go. They remind us that endings are also beginnings, and in the stillness of the colder months, the seeds of renewal are quietly preparing to sprout.

The Quiet Power of Rest

The quiet of winter offers lessons in endurance and reflection. Ancient knowledge speaks of the importance of conserving energy, seeking shelter, and finding warmth not just in the physical sense but within our connections to others and the Earth. The harshness of the season teaches resilience, while its stillness invites us to listen—to the land, to the stories of the ancestors, and to our own inner truths.

The Promise of Renewal

As spring whispers its arrival, life stirs again. The old ways teach us to watch closely—to see the first buds, hear the songs of returning birds, and feel the warming sun. This is a time for new beginnings, for planting seeds not just in the Earth but in our lives and communities. The wisdom of renewal reminds us that growth comes from nurturing both ourselves and the world around us.

Melding with Nature

Through every season, the old ways call us to slow down and reconnect. To step away from distractions and embrace the gifts of the natural world. Whether it is the fragrance of a blooming flower, the chill of snow on our skin, or the hum of bees in a summer garden, nature's rhythms offer healing and balance.

A Sacred Responsibility

The cycles of the seasons also remind us of our role as caretakers of the Earth. The wisdom of native cultures teaches that to live well, we must honor the land, respect its limits, and protect it for those yet to come. By living in harmony with nature, we not only ensure our survival but also preserve the beauty and wisdom that sustains us.

As the seasons turn, let us remember the sacred circle of life and the teachings of those who walked this land before us. In honoring the Earth, we honor ourselves and all that we are connected to.

13 SURVIVAL

There's something humbling about being in the wild. The towering trees, the endless skies, and the sounds of nature remind us of how small we are—and how connected we are to the Earth. But stepping into the wilderness isn't just an escape from the noise of daily life; it's also a reminder that survival is a skill, not a guarantee.

When I think about survival, I imagine what it would be like to rely only on what the land provides. Could I identify the right plants to eat? Would I know how to build a shelter? The truth is, nature is full of resources, but it requires respect and knowledge to use them wisely.

This chapter is about learning how to see the forest not as a challenge, but as an ally. It's about the wisdom of preparation, the creativity of survival, and the deep respect we must show to the Earth that sustains us. Let's explore how we can work with nature, not against it, and discover the tools, plants, and skills that can help us survive—and thrive—in the wild.

How to Survive in the Woods

Every year, people head into the woods to enjoy nature, and most of the time, everything is fine. But what if something unexpected happens? It's important to be prepared—not just with food and water, but also with basic survival knowledge. Knowing which plants and resources can help you survive is essential.

Always Be Prepared

Before going into the woods, make sure to pack:

- Warm Clothing: Even if it's warm during the day, it can get cold at night.
- Matches in a Waterproof Container: These can be a lifesaver.
- A First Aid Kit: Always have one handy.
- Basic Knowledge of Edible Plants and Herbs: This can make all the difference if you're lost.

If you find yourself unprepared and in a survival situation, here are some natural resources to help you.

- Edible Plants and Trees
- Pine Trees
- Needles: Boil them to make tea.
- Inner Bark: The soft, inner layer is edible.
- Young Pine Cones: These can be eaten.
- Roots: Boil young pine roots, peel the first layer, and eat the sweet inner part.
  - o Benefits: High in vitamin A, vitamin C, and beta-carotene.

Wild Garlic and Onions
- Found in temperate regions.
- Identified by their strong, characteristic smell.

Chickweed
- Common Chickweed: Has oval leaves with pointed tips and white hairs along the stem. It can be eaten raw.
- Mouse-Ear Chickweed: Needs to be boiled to remove the hairs before eating.

Burdock
- Known for its burs that stick to your clothes.
  - o Young Roots: Can be eaten.
  - o Older Roots: Very bitter but can be used to make tea.

Rose Hips
- Found in winter, easily spotted by their bright color.
- Can be eaten raw or brewed into tea. High in vitamin C.

Velvet Shank Mushrooms
- Orange caps make them easy to identify.
- Grow on dead wood, especially elm and oak trees, and usually in groups.

Nettles
- A superfood rich in protein, vitamins, and iron.
- Wear gloves when picking to avoid stings.

Acorns
- Pick ripe ones from the ground.
- Full of healthy fats.
- Soak in warm water before using.

Uses: Grind into powder to make coffee or flour.

How to Use Acorns
- Acorn Coffee: Grind the acorns into a powder, boil water, and brew like regular coffee.
- Acorn Flour: Grind the acorns into flour for cooking.

Surviving with Creativity

When you're lost in the woods, you'll need to use your imagination. The food may not be what you're used to, but it can keep you alive. And when you're rescued, you can share the story of how Mother Nature provided for you.

Being prepared and knowing how to use what's around you can make all the difference. Stay safe and remember: nature has more to offer than you might think.

In the wild, where the trees stretch toward the heavens and the earth hums with life, ancient wisdom reminds us of a simple truth: the land provides. Native cultures of the Americas understood this deeply, viewing the forest not as a challenge but as a partner in survival. The natural world, when respected, offers all that is needed for sustenance, healing, and protection.

Preparation as a Sacred Act

Just as one does not journey into life unprepared, entering the wilderness requires foresight and care. Our ancestors believed that preparation was not merely practical but also spiritual. Before stepping into the embrace of the forest, they would gather tools, knowledge, and prayers, recognizing that readiness is an offering of respect to the natural world.

Reading the Land's Signs

The wild is a teacher, but its lessons are for those who observe with open eyes and hearts. Traditional wisdom speaks of knowing the plants, trees, and waters as one knows a friend. Every leaf, root, and stream carries the potential for nourishment or healing. Yet, they also caution against haste—knowledge must guide every choice, for the land's gifts come with responsibility.

Survival Through Partnership

When lost or in need, the forest becomes a partner in survival. Roots, berries, leaves, and even bark carry the power to sustain life. Native teachings emphasize that the key to using these resources is mindfulness: take only what is needed, and always offer gratitude. In doing so, one maintains balance, ensuring that the forest remains abundant for all creatures.

Creativity and Adaptability

Survival is not just about tools or resources—it is a mindset. Ancient ways teach the importance of creativity and adaptability, of seeing opportunity where others might see scarcity. A fallen tree is shelter; a thorny plant is sustenance. The forest challenges us to think differently, to live in harmony with its rhythm.

Respect for the Land

Ultimately, the lesson of survival is a lesson in respect. The land is not an enemy to conquer but a home to honor. By walking gently, observing keenly, and taking only what is needed, we not only survive but thrive in the wilderness.

The wisdom of the Old Ways reminds us that nature is more than a backdrop—it is a partner, a teacher, and a source of life. Whether in times of ease or challenge, the forest provides for those who walk with humility and gratitude. As the elders say, "Listen to the land, and it will teach you all you need to know."

14 BACK IN THE DAY

When I think back to how people lived long ago, I'm amazed at their resourcefulness. They didn't have pharmacies, hospitals, or the internet, but they had something we often overlook—nature. Plants, roots, and herbs were their medicine, and healers dedicated their lives to understanding the gifts of the Earth.

These weren't quick fixes or shortcuts. Healing in those days required patience, rituals, and respect for the plants. Every remedy carried not just the power of the herb, but also the spirit of gratitude and connection to the natural world.

Today, we're rediscovering some of this ancient wisdom. As we do, it feels like reconnecting with something deeply human—an understanding that we are part of the Earth, not separate from it. The old ways remind us to slow down, observe, and appreciate the world around us. There's a beauty in knowing that even the simplest plant could hold the power to heal.

The Old Ways

Have you ever wondered how many plants around us have healing powers? It's like solving a giant puzzle. Out of all the plants in the world, we've only discovered a small number of their benefits.

Centuries ago, people spent their lives searching for ways to heal others. Healers worked to cure kings, queens, knights, and others of the upper class. A fascinating book called Old English Herbals by Elenore Sinclair Rohde describes how people in those times used herbs.

They were very serious about their herbal practices. They chanted songs, followed strict rituals, and believed timing was crucial for the healing to work. Sometimes the process took days, requiring repeated steps. If someone didn't follow the instructions exactly, they were told to start over. If a person healed but still felt weak, they were told their strength would return with time.

Herbs Then and Now

Some herbs used centuries ago are still used today, although their names have changed. Here are a few examples:

- Wayboard: Now known as Plantain
- Maythen: Chamomile
- Wer Gulu: Nettle
- Unfor Traedd: Knotweed
- Joy of Ground: Periwinkle

The Anglo-Saxons knew about at least 500 plants for healing. Many of these have been forgotten over time, but books like the Leech Book have preserved this knowledge.

The Leech Book: A Window to the Past

The Leech Book is one of the oldest surviving manuscripts on herbal medicine. It describes how herbs were used not only for healing people but also for protecting against "monsters," curing livestock, and treating illnesses in cattle, horses, and pigs.

Back then, pandemics were called "flying venom." Healers used a combination of nine herbs to treat people. While some remedies were helpful, others were harsh or even dangerous. Reading about those times makes us thankful for modern medicine!

Learning From the Past

Today, some of us are rediscovering the benefits of herbs. However, it's important to be cautious. Some plants look similar but are not the same. Mushrooms are a perfect example—many edible mushrooms closely resemble poisonous ones.

If you're interested in foraging for herbs, it's smart to:

- Bring a guidebook with clear pictures and descriptions.
- Learn to identify plants carefully to avoid harmful look-alikes.

A Renewed Respect for Nature

Our ancestors relied on plants for healing, protection, and survival. As we relearn these old ways, we also learn to respect the power of nature. Whether for health or history, exploring the world of herbs is a fascinating journey into the wisdom of the past.

The plants around us whisper stories of healing, survival, and balance, as they have for countless generations. Native insights from the original Americas teaches us that every living thing carries a purpose, a lesson, and a gift. In these traditions, plants are not mere resources—they are sacred relatives, interconnected with the web of life.

Healing as a Sacred Practice

For centuries, healers of the Americas understood that the power of a plant was not just in its physical properties but in its spirit. They approached healing with reverence, blending practical knowledge with ritual. Songs, prayers, and offerings often accompanied the harvest of medicinal herbs, ensuring that the balance between taking and giving back was maintained.

Like the Anglo-Saxon chants and precise rituals, these practices remind us that healing is not just about the body but also the soul and the harmony between humanity and nature.

Plants as Teachers

Indigenous wisdom often speaks of plants as teachers. The Cedar, Sage, Tobacco, and Sweetgrass of the North carry lessons of purification, prayer, and connection. In the South, plants like Ayahuasca and Coca are revered for their ability to teach resilience, reflection, and healing. To those who listen, each plant offers a message unique to its place in the ecosystem.

The practice of learning from plants requires patience, humility, and respect—qualities modern life often rushes us to forget. Like the careful study of the Leech Book or Anglo-Saxon remedies, indigenous healers remind us to observe with care and seek wisdom with gratitude.

Renewing the Old Ways in a Modern World

As we rediscover herbal knowledge, we must also remember the humility of our ancestors. Foraging, cultivating, and using plants requires responsibility—not just to our health but to the land that provides these gifts. The guidance of tribal traditions, like carrying a modern guidebook for foraging, offers protection against misuse and deepens our respect for the natural world.

Harmony and Gratitude

The Old Ways remind us that healing is not a solo journey—it is a path of relationship. When a plant heals us, it asks for nothing but gratitude in return. In honoring these exchanges, we learn not just about herbs but about the interconnectedness of life itself.

May we walk this path with the wisdom of those who came before, honoring the sacred relationship between humans and the natural world. For in the leaves, roots, and flowers lies not just medicine for the body, but also healing for the spirit.

As the elders say, "The Earth does not belong to us; we belong to the Earth." So, let us tend this ancient knowledge with care, walking gently and learning always.

ABOUT THE AUTHOR

Juanita Holaday is a Natural Alternative Specialist, holistic herbalist, Reiki healer, and cofounder of the Natural Alternative Specialist program at St. Paul's Free University. With years of experience in alternative health sciences, Juanita has dedicated her career to empowering others through the integration of ancient wisdom and modern health practices.

As the youngest in a multi-generational lineage of Curanderos, shamans, and natural healers, Juanita carries forward her family's legacy of service to the world. She combines her deep connection to ancestral knowledge with advanced training in herbal remedies, energy healing, and holistic health coaching.

Juanita's groundbreaking work has helped countless individuals embrace natural solutions for their health challenges. Now retired, she enjoys sharing her knowledge through writing and workshops, helping others find balance, vitality, and joy in their lives. Solutions from My Ancestors for Everyday Health Problems is her heartfelt offering to all seeking a path to natural wellness.

For more information, visit juanitaholaday.com.

* 9 7 9 8 7 1 5 0 9 1 2 4 6 *